Praise for *Hearing Maud*

This is an extraordinary and poignant memoir written in an embodied and attentive style. White offers us glimpses of global deaf history woven with the tapestry of her own life/story and accentuated with the lives of Rosa and Maud Praed. *Hearing Maud* is a literary seduction about literary seductions.

Brenda Jo Brueggemann
Lend Me Your Ear* and *Deaf Subjects

In her three-part soliloquy on her search for belonging, understanding and love, Jessica White achieves an extraordinarily accomplished fusion of personal memoir, biography and deaf studies. White's searching ruminations about the implications of her lifelong deafness together with her scholarly research of Maud Praed – the deaf daughter of nineteenth-century Queensland expatriate novelist Rosa Praed – and dive into deaf studies resound with tension, drama and insight without yielding to sentiment or polemic. By navigating Maud's heartbreaking story of being deaf in the late nineteenth and early twentieth centuries, White locates her own personal Australian experiences of growing up deaf within the panorama of deaf history. In doing so, she not only arrives at an enriched understanding of her deaf self, but also provides a uniquely Australian contribution to the literature of, about and by deaf people.

Donna McDonald
The Art of Being Deaf: A Memoir* and *Jack's Story

In *Hearing Maud* Jessica White fulfils, with grace, elegance and a fierce regard for truth-telling, writing's primary task: to tell it as it is; but as no one has ever told it before. This is a book of wonder. It gives voice to silence.

Martin Edmond
Battarbee and Namatjira* and *Isinglass

HEARING MAUD

Jessica White was raised in north-west New South Wales and, at age four, lost most of her hearing from meningitis. An avid reader and writer, she journeyed from her country school of 100 pupils to publishing her first novel at age twenty-nine, before graduating with a PhD from the University of London. Her first novel, *A Curious Intimacy*, was published in 2007. It won a *Sydney Morning Herald* Best Young Novelist award, was shortlisted for the Western Australian Premier's award and the Dobbie award for a first book by a woman writer, and longlisted for the international IMPAC award. Her second novel, *Entitlement*, was published in 2012. Jessica is the recipient of funding from Arts Queensland and the Australia Council for the Arts, and she has been selected for residencies in Tasmania and the Australia Council's BR Whiting Studio in Rome. Her short fiction, poetry and essays have appeared in Australian and international literary journals, including *Review of Australian Fiction*, *Overland, Island*, *Griffith Review*, *Westerly* and *Southerly*. Jessica is an academic at The University of Queensland where she is writing an ecobiography of Georgiana Molloy, Western Australia's first female scientist. She lives in Brisbane with her partner and a coterie of plants that she tries to keep alive, and she can be found at www.jessicawhite.com.au.

HEARING MAUD

JESSICA WHITE

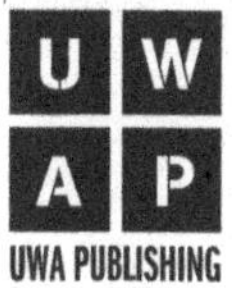

First published in 2019 and reprinted 2020 by
UWA Publishing
Crawley, Western Australia 6009
www.uwap.uwa.edu.au

UWAP is an imprint of UWA Publishing,
a division of The University of Western Australia.

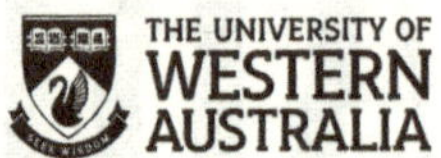

ISBN: 978-1-76080-038-3

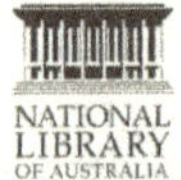

A catalogue record for this book is available from the National Library of Australia

Cover design by Alissa Dinallo
Cover image: Maud Praed, State Library of NSW
Typeset by J&M Typesetting
Printed by McPherson's Printing Group

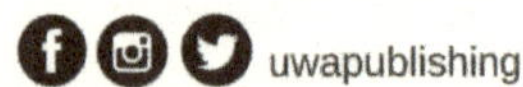

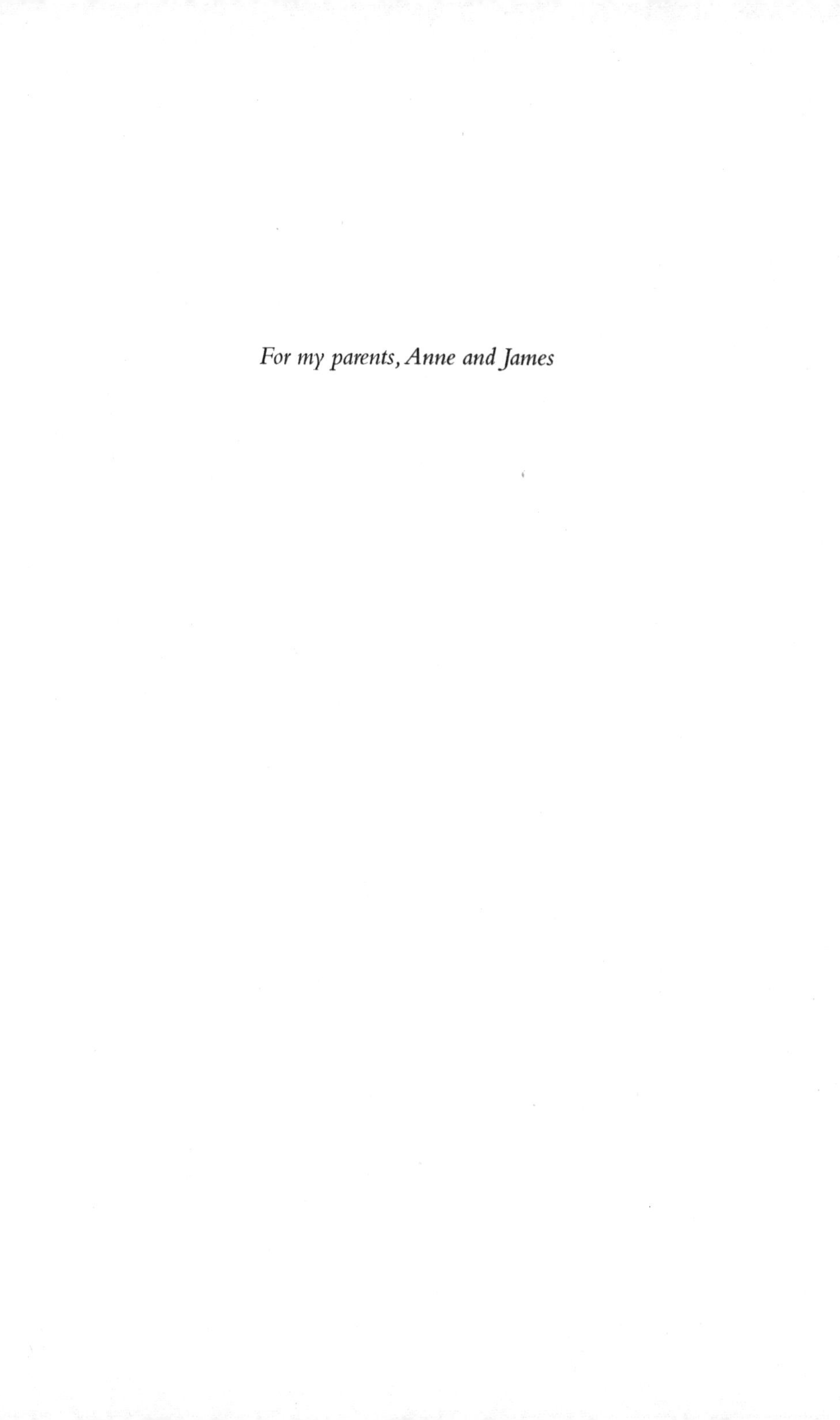

For my parents, Anne and James

Contents

Prologue

A Poison and a Cure

On a morning in early summer, I lay on a pale-blue trampoline beneath the apricot tree. Its branches, which scraped against my bedroom window in storms, arched over me. The tree was planted by workmen who had lived in our weatherboard cottage before my parents moved in, but it never bore fruit.

My mother appeared at the side of the trampoline.

'How are you feeling?' she asked.

I shook my head, unable to answer. I was nearly four years old. My head, neck and shoulders were awash with an ache. A light breeze scraped my skin like a blade, while the sunlight, normally soft and dappled, speared through the leaves above.

My mother sensed there was something wrong, she would tell me in later years, something worse than the flu. She thought for a few minutes, then went inside and changed her farm clothes for a skirt and blouse. She collected her handbag, found my shoes and scrawled a note for my father.

Back at the trampoline, she wriggled the shoes onto my feet. 'We're going to town to see the doctor.'

'Okay.' It was hard to speak.

Mum collected my brother and sister, Oliver and Bella, and dropped them at my grandmother's house a few kilometres away. We then drove over rough gravel roads for forty minutes until we reached Gunnedah. When the local doctor saw me, his movements became quick and urgent: I was to go to Tamworth Base Hospital immediately. Mum drove for another hour. Sweat formed beneath her hands, making the steering wheel sticky.

At the hospital she watched in horror as she held me down while I screamed and the doctor drove a needle into my spine. Results confirmed it was meningitis and I was given a massive dose of antibiotics to kill the infection on the lining of my brain. After that there was nothing to do but wait.

A few hours later my father arrived. My godparents, who lived on a property on the way to Tamworth, rushed in. They sat by the bedside in the darkness while I had a respiratory arrest and stopped breathing. A minister appeared, praying silently with my godparents, who were devout Christians. My atheist parents, having lost a child five years before, held hands against the death of this one.

In the morning, my eyes opened. The adults held their breath. I blinked: ever combative, I had won.

I was in hospital for a month. My bed was adjacent to a sliding glass door that led to a small, fenced courtyard. If kids wet their beds, nurses slung the sheets over the fence to dry. Sometimes those sheets were mine and the nurses chided me for it.

My father often sat beside me, reading from a picture book about Strawberry Shortcake. I twisted the plastic identification bracelet on my wrist, unable to follow what was happening because his voice was a low burble. I liked the pictures, though.

Finally, I was allowed to go home. I tucked my stuffed toys, Mr Tickle and Mr Chatterbox, into the car seat beside me.

Within a few weeks, my parents realised something wasn't right.

'She keeps asking me what I'm saying,' my mother said. 'This morning I yelled at her down the verandah to clean her teeth and she just looked at me.'

I leaned against the doorway in the kitchen, watching them. My father laid his hand on my head and stroked my hair.

Some weeks later, he and I rose in the coal-glow of morning and set off for Sydney, a six-hour drive away. We stopped for lunch by the banks of a river and took out the sandwiches Mum had made. A weeping willow drooped into the water. Beyond it was a rickety wooden bridge, over which cars sometimes rattled. The sunlight was bright, the grassy bank warm beneath our legs. When crumbs from the sandwiches fell into the water, a swathe of eels appeared.

'Do they bite?' I asked.

'They can do.'

'Will I fall in?'

'No.'

The bank looked precipitous and the eels writhing below our feet were disturbing. I drew up my legs.

In Sydney we stayed with friends who lived in an apartment, the first one I'd ever seen. Their kids, a boy and girl, showed me how to slide down the carpeted flight of stairs between each floor. In the evening, we put on a finger puppet show for the adults, who drank gin and tonics in the living room. I couldn't follow what the kids were saying and quickly lost the thread of my lines. I kneeled beside the cardboard stage, silent and ashamed.

This sense of soreness, of being around people and not knowing how to deal with them, has throbbed all my life. This is my first recollection of the feeling, and yet I have no memory of the visit to the audiologist who found I had lost all the hearing in my left ear and half in my right.

It transpired that the large dose of antibiotics injected to cure the infection on the lining of my brain had saved me, but it had also damaged the nerves of my cochlea. My life came to be defined by what the ancient Greeks termed a *pharmakon*, that which is a poison and a cure.

Beyond the windows of my apartment, it's a brilliant Brisbane day. The palm tree, which harbours orchids in its hairy bark, sways in the breeze. My desk is smothered in handwritten drafts, typed copies, photocopies of articles, a 1904 edition of a novel titled *Nyria* and a copy of a small photograph. It shows a young woman wearing a well-fitted coat, a lace cravat and a large woollen hat with a velvet flower. She looks away from the lens with heavy-lidded eyes, her mouth open as if to speak. This is Maud Praed, the deaf daughter of Rosa Praed, a nineteenth-century expatriate Australian novelist.

As a writer, it's my job to go into the underworld, to collect the stories of the dead and bring them back to the living. When I uncovered Maud's story I realised that deafness, too, could be a poison and a cure, and that the way the pendulum swung in favour of one or the other depended on the time and culture in which the deaf person lived. For Maud, it was a bane, a word from the Old English word *bana* meaning 'thing causing death'. Except that

Maud didn't die until she was sixty-seven, kept away from those she loved, her presence a footnote in her famous mother's life.

For me, deafness led to writing, which assuaged my persistent loneliness and gave me a sense of purpose. It also led me to Rosa and Maud. Through them, I learned that I had been assimilated into the world of hearing people and that the deaf part of myself had been ghosted, to the point where no one knew that I was deaf until I told them, to the point where I barely even knew it myself.

Now, in the bright light at my desk, I hold a pen in one hand, the stories from the underworld in the other. I begin to write.

1

Be/Longing

I step off the tram, struggling to remember the map I'd loaded on the internet before I left my friend's house. It's the end of winter and wet brown leaves spread over the road. Before me are the cream sandstone buildings of the University of Melbourne. I wander through the gates and, to my relief, find the administration block. My anxiety about being late subsides.

I introduce myself to a receptionist. 'I'm here for the scholarship interview.'

'Head up the stairs. There's a chair outside the door. If you wait there, someone will collect you.'

The stairs creak underfoot. I come from a family of performers and I know how to act, but my pulse still patters faster than usual.

At the top I find the chair and settle into it, knitting my fingers together.

'Jessica?' A woman in a dark jacket and skirt opens the heavy wooden door.

I stand, my body leaning forward in anticipation.

'I'm part of your interviewing panel. Come through. We turned down the heaters so you can hear. They were rattling a bit.'

A long-limbed man and a woman with dark, bobbed hair sit at the table. I pull out a chair opposite. I'm glad the interviewers are close enough for me to hear them without straining.

'Tell us why you'd like to go to the London Consortium.' The woman with dark hair clasps her hands on the table.

'A few years ago I went on exchange to Berkeley at the University of California. It was so amazing that I want to study overseas again. My brother's in England and I'd like to join him. The PhD program is also rigorous and multidisciplinary, which suits me because I write both literary criticism and creative works.'

'You've been writing a novel?'

'Yes, through my Masters. I could have gone straight to a PhD after I finished Honours, but if I did that I wouldn't have finished the book.'

'How's it going?'

'I write a couple of thousand words a day, but I throw most of it out.'

'That's a lot of writing!'

I shrug. 'I like socialising but it's difficult because I can't hear, so I have to find other things to do, like reading and writing.'

The thin man speaks but I don't catch all of it because it's hard for me to hear lower pitches. I piece together what I've heard and his sentence unfurls. 'How much hearing do you have?'

'About twenty-five per cent. I was speaking by the time I got meningitis so my parents sent me to a mainstream school. People usually don't know that I'm deaf until I tell them.'

'I teach audiology,' he adds.

'Ah, I see.'

'What do you want to research in London?'

'Literary seductions. The way you can draw someone closer through writing.'

'Interesting.'

'Have you been in touch with the office about having your flights to Melbourne reimbursed?' My attention swerves back to the woman in the suit.

'No, that wasn't mentioned to me.' I contemplate adding that I didn't want to do a phone interview because my anxiety about listening on phones can make me abrupt and terse, but I don't want to use my disability as an excuse. 'I thought it was important to come.'

At the close of the interview the audiology lecturer says, 'The problem with people like you is that you make deafness look easy.'

I look at his angular face, and my shoulders sag with relief. This tall, spare man has understood the years of standing by myself against a wall because I don't know how to start a conversation; the days of picking up one book after another to alleviate my loneliness; the hours of speech therapy and coaching in small talk.

'Thank you.' I shake his hand and walk out. Even if I never win the scholarship, it has been worth coming all that way just to hear his words.

Back in Sydney, I continue the dull administrative job I've taken on to save money for London. The office ceiling is oppressively low, but large windows look out to the Downing Centre Court on Elizabeth Street. The court had once been Mark Foy's department store and the words 'Hats', 'Trimmings' and 'Scarves' stretch across the top of the building in a mosaic of green and orange tiles.

On the eastern side is the lush greenness of Hyde Park, to which I often escape at lunch.

I stand at the photocopier, absently placing originals on the glass and pressing the Start button. My job is to write letters to people about their unpaid parking fines. Glum with boredom, I gaze about the office. In an effort to ward off claustrophobia, I've brightened my workspace with an elephant fern, a row of books and photos of my friends. It looks like an oasis.

Nearby, a young Asian man leans over a desk, reading the sports section of the newspaper. I know his name is Alex, but that's all. He wears a pale-blue checked shirt and well-pressed navy trousers. His waist is trim. I wonder, idly, what it would be like to rest my hands on his hips.

Later that day, I approach his desk with a trivial question about some paperwork. He chats to a colleague next to him but I can't hear their conversation. When he notices me waiting, he swivels around. 'Yes, ma'am?'

I'm delighted. No one has called me *ma'am* before.

He emails to ask for help with something he's written. Although his written English is poor, his wit sparkles through. I scold him for his bad grammar. Lust travels into the wires of the network.

A lover once gave me a copy of Frances Wilson's *Literary Seductions: Compulsive Writers and Diverted Readers.* Although our relationship soured suddenly, his inscription charmed me: *Dear Jessica, I saw this book on the shelves and was instantly reminded of you and your words. l. X (your diverted reader).*

'In literary seductions words become flesh,' Wilson writes. 'Rather than being captivated by a smile, a voice, or a gesture it is in the pattern of certain letters, the positions of particular vowels, the flow of the sounds or the story that the lover drowns.'[1]

All day, amidst the tedium of our work, Alex and I email banter, admonishment and jokes. Sometimes his wit trips me and I, unused to being tripped, pick myself up from the floor, laughing. As well as his words, I'm entranced by his brown eyes, the tattoo of his name in a character – it's Vietnamese, I find – on his right biceps, his narrow wrists and thick black hair. I imagine what it would feel like to touch it: dark water falling through my fingers.

I invite him to watch *The Incredible Hulk* at Fox Studios. I arrive early, and to pass the time I wander into a bookstore near the cinema and examine the bookshelves. I pull out a copy of Simon Winchester's *Krakatoa: The Day the World Exploded*, about a volcano that erupted in the nineteenth century. I read a few pages, but the prose is dull.

I check my watch and head to the cinema, and Alex soon arrives. The movie bores me because I can't hear it, but I'm alert to Alex shifting in his seat, the sharp smell of his aftershave. He drives me home but doesn't kiss me.

We spend more time together at work, eating lunch in the overblown green of Hyde Park, lying on our backs to watch a seagull in the sky, a tiny dot soaring among clouds. Or we head to cheap Asian takeaway joints. At the rickety plastic table in Kim's Thai, he slides a pair of chopsticks from their thin paper sleeve. 'It's funny that they've given us these to eat with. Usually Thais eat with a fork and spoon.'

His phone rings. He checks the number on the screen.

'Sorry, I have to take this, it's my Dad.'

As Alex chats, I watch people ordering food, handing over money, reaching for warm plastic containers over the counter and nodding their thanks. I hear a rustle of strange sounds, round and hollow, and turn my attention to Alex's lips. For some reason I can't read what he's saying. A second later it dawns: he's switched to Vietnamese.

I'm ashamed of my surprise. Of course he's bilingual; I just never thought to look past his broad Australian accent.

A few weeks after our first conversation, Alex knocks on the door of my Art Deco apartment in Randwick. My flatmates are out that night.

His hand slides over my backside as I lead him to my room. I grab his wrist. 'Wait.'

'What is it?'

On my desk, in a pool of rose-coloured light cast by my lamp, lies a letter from the University of Melbourne.

'I won the scholarship. I'm going to London.'

'That's amazing! Congratulations.' He pulls me to him, holding me tight. But, I later think, not tightly enough.

I push him onto the bed, sit astride him and pull off my T-shirt, unhook my bra.

'You're beautiful.' His face is soft with pleasure.

I bend down, kissing him to hide my sadness.

I am twenty-five and this is the first time I've had unfettered access to a man's body. Before this had been awkward fumbling with a boy in the narrow bed in my residential college at the University of Wollongong. When it became apparent to him that I wasn't interested, he put a sign on his door that said 'Virgin Violator', although, when he'd slipped his fingers into me, he'd said, 'There's nothing there.'

'Yeah, it broke a while ago.' I didn't know how. It might have been when I had thrush, or from exercise.

A year later, I took my clothes off with a man who loved reading and who gave me *Literary Seductions*. Later, he suggested a ménage à trois. This was too much for a young, naïve woman from the country. I ended our liaison.

With this smooth, brown-skinned boy, I fall like Alice into Wonderland. On the hour-long walk to work past Centennial Park and the Sydney Cricket Ground, I listen to ABBA and imagine my hands sweeping down the hard arch of his back. There's a small bump on his right arm, a chicken pox scar. When I stroke his arm, my fingers linger on the smooth, raised skin.

Occasionally I remember the scholarship letter, the plane ticket I need to book, the savings I need to transfer, but I let them fade, murmuring under my breath to 'Dancing Queen'. I walk through the cramped but colourful streets of Surry Hills, passing homeless men sitting outside a bakery on milk crates, and workers carrying cups of coffee. As I approach the office, my step becomes springier.

Inside, I wave hello to Alex, log on and check my workload, then open my email. *How was your evening?*

The day begins.

He fucks me on the carpet so hard I laugh. Downstairs lives Neville, a devout Christian who tacks Christmas cards to his front door. I have no doubt he can hear us.

'I love you,' I say.

'You shouldn't.'

I stop smiling. My back stings. Later I discover a large strip of skin has peeled off, leaving it red and raw. I pick at the scab for weeks.

My anxiety gathers, a rustle of bees round my head.

'I don't know why I'm going to London.'

'You'll be fine. It's just a walk in the park for you.'

'I wish I wasn't leaving.'

There's no answer.

I sit on his desk in a short skirt. He reaches between my legs to open his drawer and take out a gift. I smile; I like getting presents.

Inside the wrapping paper is a case, and inside the case, a silver pen. My smile broadens as I turn it in my hands, then I read the inscription with a quick intake of air. *Walk in the Park.*

The night before I leave for England, I'm in his bed. I smell rain outside, but I can't hear anything.

'Is it raining?' I'm hopeful, my head against his chest.

'Yeah. It's annoying.'

I laugh, closing my eyes. As a child, I'd loved falling asleep to the sound of rain on a corrugated-iron roof. Growing up on a dry property where my father's constant checking of the gauge inflamed my anxiety, rain meant security. I imagined it seeping into the soil, swelling grains of wheat until they split open, their heads stretching up to the light.

In Alex's arms, I'm wrapped in my pea-green doona again, listening to the old gum tree on the front lawn shaking rain from its hair.

But it's time to go.

Outside in the chilly air, he puts his sheepskin jacket around my shoulders and drives me across the harbour to my friend's house in North Sydney. He takes my hand as we cross the road.

'Did you remember your earrings? They were on the ironing board.'

I slip my hand into my pocket and feel the thin, silver fish. 'Yes, I've got them.'

I press the intercom to my friend's flat, then lean towards Alex for a last kiss. The door clicks open and I break away. The next day I board the flight to London, leaving him behind.

These days, when I walk along the Brisbane River in the evening, passing dogs and sweaty joggers, I imagine what would have happened if I hadn't won the scholarship. I might have married him and had two kids with sleek hair. Or I might have become restless and walked away.

Instead, my passion erupted and spilled, burning runnels into our history.

I land at Heathrow in the morning, numb with tiredness, but my spirits lift when I see Oliver waiting in the crowd. He lives in a village named Malmesbury, fifty kilometres east of Bristol. He doesn't take me there immediately, because the first rule of jet lag, I'm to find after many flights between England and Australia, is never to sleep during the day.

We drive to Castle Combe, an exquisite medieval village through which a clear stream burbles. Outside a whitewashed pub, a lady sells small, handmade bags. I pick up one tufted with brown fur, and run my fingers over it. I like touching things, and I can tell what I'm looking for in my wardrobe by the feel of the fabric.

My sensitivity to touch is related to my deafness. When the brain is deprived of information from one sense, it often compensates by processing input from another. This is known as 'cross-modal plasticity.' There are a large number of anecdotal reports of people who have lost one of their senses and show an extraordinary ability with one or more of their remaining senses. The French writer Diderot, for example, described the famous case of a blind mathematician who could recognise fake from real coins by touching them.[2] Research shows that some deaf people have enhanced motion detection, visual orienting, and attention in their peripheral vision.[3] This makes sense, as people who sign need to focus on the movement of hands and faces. Others might need to pick up activity in the corner of their eye, such as a motorbike coming towards them, which they might not hear.

'How about I buy that handbag for you, Jess?' Oliver asks. 'A welcome-to-England present.'

'Yes!'

We take tea and scones in the Manor House and wander through the immaculate gardens. In the pleasure of seeing Oliver again and the novelty of being in a new place, my thoughts of Alex recede.

During the week at Oliver's, I struggle to keep warm. It's autumn and the air is damp. I walk through Malmesbury's narrow, cobbled streets until I reach its edge, where stone cottages are bordered by fields of thick, wet grass. I turn back and head for the abbey. In the graveyard, a headstone tells the story of a girl who was killed by a tiger in 1703.

'It can't be true,' I say to Oliver when he comes home from work.

'It is. She was a barmaid at the White Lion pub. The tiger was in a circus that stopped by. She kept aggravating the tiger, so it got annoyed and killed her.'

I don't know whether to be amused or horrified.

Then the week is over and I catch the train to London, where

I've arranged to live in a college for postgraduate students. The college's manager has put me in a room near the entrance of the building in case there's a fire and I don't hear the alarm and someone has to get me out. The room is a cell, its one barred window opening to the brick wall and pipes of the adjacent building. I put down my suitcase, my happiness of the previous week draining like water down a plughole.

In 1998, when I was twenty, I sat before another interviewing panel, this one at the University of Wollongong where I was doing my undergraduate degree. Before me was a woman from the Study Abroad office and an American man. My academic transcript lay between us.

At the Study Abroad information meeting we had been advised, 'Don't bother applying to go to Berkeley. Everyone wants to go to Berkeley, but they only take the very best and most people don't get in.'

I relayed this comment to Mum over the phone.

'Rubbish,' she replied. 'Berkeley is the top university. Of course you should apply to go there.'

At the interviewing table, the American man asked me, 'You want to be a writer?'

'Yes.'

'You have distinctions and high distinctions for all of your subjects, except these two writing subjects in your first year, for which you have credits. Why is that?'

'Writing is a craft. It takes a long time to become good at it.'

He smiled. 'Thank you. That's the answer I was looking for.'

I was accepted into Berkeley and I won a scholarship to help with my costs while I was there.

As my departure date drew near I packed and repacked my backpack, then my parents drove me to Sydney. At the airport, nervous and awkward, we drank coffee while Mum relayed the steps I needed to follow to get through Customs, Immigration and then onto the plane itself. This was the first time I'd been overseas on my own, and I was petrified that I wouldn't hear the overhead announcements and would miss the plane.

When my parents said goodbye, my mother's eyes were red with tears. I was alarmed; it was the first time I'd ever seen her cry.

I made it on board, but the plane was delayed on the tarmac for an hour. I couldn't hear the captain's announcements so I gathered courage to ask the woman next to me what he was saying.

'There's a problem with the engine that they're checking.' Her American accent startled me. Of course, I reminded myself, I'm on my way to the United States. She offered me some sweets from the packet she'd opened but I shook my head, too agitated to eat.

As the flight was delayed, I missed my connecting flight from Los Angeles. By the time I finally reached San Francisco, I hadn't eaten anything except a packet of crackers over twenty-four hours. I found a hotel and food and slept. When I woke fourteen hours later, it was as though I'd shed a layer of myself.

On the gorgeous campus, centred by Sather Tower, a tall campanile clad in Sierra White granite, I found myself among confident American students who were never afraid to express their thoughts. In this place, it was normal to be different, to be an intellectual and a workaholic, and my deafness didn't matter. It was also expected that one should have opinions. In class, we were graded on participation. I was desperate for straight As, so I put my hand up and began to speak.

All my life, my family have spoken up or spoken out to make sure I was getting the same opportunities as everyone else. When I was fifteen, we moved to the town of Armidale. At the cinema one evening, my mother pushed to the front of queue so that we could ensure we accessed the seat that was best for hearing the loop system. This is a piece of wire that runs around the walls of a cinema and transmits a magnetic signal to my hearing aid. When I switch my hearing aid to the 'telecoil' or 'T' switch, it picks up the signal from the wire (which carries the sound from the movie) and cuts out any background noise. When the system works, the sound is clear and I can hear well. Usually, however, it doesn't. In this cinema, it was next to hopeless, so it was important to sit in the right place.

'Excuse me,' said the woman already at the front of the queue, her tone sharp with annoyance, 'but we were here first.'

'My daughter's deaf,' Mum explained. 'We need to make sure we can get a seat that she can hear in.'

The woman pressed her lips together and turned away. I loathed the tension and I loathed myself for causing it. I would rather have missed the film.

In America, there was no one to speak for me. My father's axiom, 'If you get chucked in the deep end, you have to swim,' turned out to be true. I shoved my fear against the wall. Who cared if I was odd? I wasn't going to be in America forever.

I was often lost as I wandered around, and discovered that a friendly smile made strangers willing to give me directions. I remembered lessons my parents gave me on making small talk when they were trying to teach me conversational skills.

'You can start with the weather.'

'But *why*? It's boring. I don't want to know about the weather. I can just look out the window.'

I began to initiate hesitant conversations about the way California's sunshine was so like Sydney's and people began to talk back. Gradually, I worked out that small talk was an icebreaker, necessary to make a path through cold and intimidating territory.

At the end of my year away, I walked out of Arrivals in Sydney Airport with a grin on my face. On the inside of my calf was a tattoo of a woman holding a spear, which I'd had done when travelling with friends in the European summer break. My mother and brother were waiting for me, arms outstretched.

'Nice mark on your leg, Jess,' Mum commented.

'It was a spur-of-the-moment thing, in Amsterdam.'

'Were you on anything?'

'No!'

It was a symbol of who I'd become: a shy and frightened girl transformed into an outspoken, although not quite fearless, woman.

Now I wanted another challenge. I liked the bustle of big cities and I was sure that a few years in London would be amazing.

That assumption was wrong.

~

The London Consortium hosts an orientation day in an elegant, light-filled room in the Institute of Contemporary Arts, which perches on a corner of St James's Park. One can stand outside the entrance to this building, look down the street and see Buckingham Palace at the end of it. For the whole time that I live in London, this never fails to delight me.

The London Consortium is a collaboration between Birkbeck College (part of the University of London), the Tate galleries, the Architectural Association and the Institute of Contemporary Arts.

Later, it expands to include the Wellcome Collection, a museum and library centred on medicine, science and art. Surrounded by artists and architects in the loud and airy room, I panic. My undergraduate degrees are in creative writing and English, and my Masters degree is also in writing. I've never been among people who don't deal with words.

I feel as I did at preschool, in a room clustered with bodies that didn't smell of the washing powder my mother and aunts used, missing the comfort of my brother who had been put into a separate room. Outside, the street was quiet, looking out to the local hospital. The houses in that street were neat, with small backyards. To someone raised in acres of space, they had seemed too close together.

A few years ago, I told Mum how much I had disliked preschool, even though I only went once a week, on Wednesdays.

'You must remember, you'd just had a major shock from the meningitis. Things were difficult for you.'

I hadn't liked being made to nap after lunch when I wanted to be running around. Instead I lay awake, watching the ceiling fan turn. Sometimes I rolled onto my side to watch my cousin Naomi sleeping. She was born one month and two days before me. Around us stretched the bodies of other kids on thin mattresses. I was bored, hot and uncomfortable.

I did, however, settle enough to enjoy painting. We pulled on billowy cotton smocks, placed our easels against a wooden fence, and dashed paint upon them.

'Very good,' my mother said when I took home my creation, wrinkled from watery paint on cheap butcher's paper.

Mr Tony, who would become my disability support teacher when I started school, visited the preschool. It was 1982. He wore a short-sleeved shirt with a tie, shorts and long white socks pulled up to his calves. In play he chased me through large cement tunnels and around the swings. I was anxious rather than amused: was I playing well enough? Was I like the other children? Was I being normal? Without my siblings and cousins around me, I felt alien. Interacting with other people seemed to hurt my skin, just as it is hurting now, in the light-filled room at the Institute of Contemporary Arts.

I take a glass of wine and glance at a man next to me. His pleasant face makes me confident enough to introduce myself. He's a polite, self-effacing Englishman studying the novelist George Orwell. Listening to his clever humour, my panic lessens to a simmer. Perhaps I won't be so completely alone in London.

As soon as I'm back in my tiny room that evening, I check my emails. There's nothing from Alex.

In one of the elegant rooms of the British Library, I wake from a nap, lifting my head from the desk. Around me, at long wooden tables, rows of readers are bent to their books, their hair illuminated by the glow of desk lamps. The ceilings are high above my head, the woodwork panelling of the walls rich and dark. I feel groggy. Although I've now been in London for a month, it still seems like a bad dream, and I'm not entirely sure what I'm doing in this cavernous room of industrious workers.

I stare blearily at the book before me, *With Fond Regards: Private Lives Through Letters*. It's a selection of letters from the National Library of Australia, edited by Elizabeth Riddell, a poet and journalist. It includes missives penned by Joseph Banks, a botanist on board James Cook's voyage to Australia; convict woman Margaret Catchpole; Jewish internees detained in Hay internment camp during the Second World War; and literary figures such as Vance and Nettie Palmer, Patrick White and Rosa Praed.

I pause at Rosa's name. I had come across it a few years before when I was researching my first novel, *A Curious Intimacy*. I'd picked up Debra Adelaide's *A Bright and Fiery Troop*, a collection of essays on nineteenth-century Australian women writers, to get a sense of their lives and writing. Rosa was featured in it.

Ever since I read *Jane Eyre* when I was supposed to be studying for my final high school exams, I have loved the fearless women of the nineteenth century. Instead of memorising equations or lines from *King Lear*, I was carried across wintry fields by Jane's passion. A year later, at the University of Wollongong, I studied nineteenth-century women writers and fell for Rachel Henning, who emigrated from England to Australia, settling in Exmoor in Queensland in 1862. She adored the fresh air and a good gallop. These women weren't designed for drawing rooms, and I liked watching how they asserted themselves in spaces where they were told they ought not go. This was one of the reasons I set my first novel in this era.

I turn to the introduction Riddell wrote to contextualise Rosa's letter. Rosa was born in 1851 at Bromelton, not far from what is now Beaudesert in Queensland. She was educated by her mother, then she married an Englishman at age twenty-one and lived with him on Curtis Island off the coast of Rockhampton. A few years later they emigrated to England, where their marriage came asunder. In its wake, Rosa met and connected with Nancy Harward, a medium. 'Rosa's life was pure melodrama,' Riddell writes. 'For every high there was a low and she died alone and lonely in 1935, her three sons dead before her, her daughter in an asylum, and herself a paragraph or two in essays by academics on

Australian literature.'[4] I sit up. As someone who has often stood on the edges of conversations, trying to listen and participate, I am sympathetic towards people who are overlooked, particularly if they are women writers.

The part of my hearing that survived is in the upper registers, so I hear women's voices more clearly than men's. This means there is less confusion and less chance of mishearing when I listen to women, and of being mocked if I don't catch something. When I learned of feminism at university, my affinity with women's voices became an obsession. I particularly identified with their historical efforts to find a voice and to have that voice published in a world that was hostile to them. As Virginia Woolf, with her ever-elegant turn of phrase, wrote in *Room of One's Own*: 'One can measure the opposition that was in the air to a woman writing when one finds that even a woman with a great turn for writing has brought herself to believe that to write a book was to be ridiculous.'[5]

I turn the page of Riddell's book and read Rosa's letter. It's written from London to her stepmother Nora in Australia at the outbreak of the First World War, but its account of German spies doesn't interest me. I load the British Library's catalogue listing under 'Praed, Rosa Caroline'. It shows some fifty works published between 1880 and 1931. I order the first of these, her novel *An Australian Heroine*. When my online account tells me the book has arrived from storage, I collect the original 1880 edition from the issue desk and carry it carefully back to my seat.

The story on those thick, creamy pages follows the pattern of Rosa's life: the heroine Esther moves from a remote island to London after marrying George, with whom she is incompatible. There was 'an utter dearth of subjects of mutual sympathy between them. George had no great acquaintance with literature, and no feeling for art, or enthusiasm for the subjective interests of life. The abstract side of existence, which had a greater interest for Esther than common-place realities, was to George a sealed book.'[6] Esther's disappointment with marriage and her sense of being shackled is a theme, I soon find, to which Rosa returned again and again.

I rub my eyes, my head too woolly to do any more reading. I make a note of the letter and the book, pack up my laptop and step outside into the grey, bitter day. The sky is overcast and the chilly air bites my skin. With no sun, there are no shadows to ground the buildings, or even myself. After a lifetime of bright Australian sunshine and a shadow reliably attached to my feet, it feels peculiar.

I wave down the bus and sit upstairs. I enjoy the novelty of red double-deckers, the way they sway around corners, the passengers stepping on and off, the doors beeping inoffensively as they open and close

With a start I realise I'm at Paddington Station. I press the bell and trundle off, heading for Talbot Square. Even after several weeks, I'm still distressed by the relentless cold that eats into my thin Australian coat, the pollution that darkens the buildings, and the monotonous clouds pressing upon everything. They dampen the air and bead on my woollen jumpers. I pass patients from the nearby hospital and people with tight, grim faces. They are buttoned up, closed in and difficult to read. No one makes eye contact, or offers a smile. I open the door to my room, drop my satchel onto the floor and start to cry.

After a spate of applications, I find a part-time job as an assistant at University College London (UCL) library, issuing books to borrowers. To get to work, I walk down Marylebone Road past Madame Tussauds, the Royal Academy of Music and the carefully tended gardens of Regent's Park, then turn into a warren of streets. I walk everywhere because I'm putting on weight and I'm trying to make my savings last. My scholarship covers my fees, but it's up to me to provide my living expenses.

I hadn't given enough thought to what London would be like. In Sydney, I'd enjoyed sitting in cafés with a book, watching people walk by and noting their shoes, sunglasses and handbags. I liked the outdoor bars, the violently green parks, the arc of impossibly blue sky overhead. As London was a big city, too, it never occurred to me that I wouldn't like it.

Having finished reading Rosa's first novel, *An Australian Heroine*, in the British Library, I realise that Rosa must have had a shock, too. Her protagonist Esther muses, 'This was not the London she had pictured to herself. She had expected to see a city of palaces and brightness, with streets filled with gaily dressed ladies in carriages with champing horses...but the low thoroughfares near the river were meaner in appearance than any colonial town. There was an air of squalor and dirt over everything, and the people she saw were rough, ill clad, and shivering.'[7]

I turn onto Gower Street, wait for the lights to change, then cross to the wide, paved courtyard of University College London. I peel off my coat as I enter the building, heading upstairs to the library. I say hello to the security guard, a kind Scottish man who wears long cardigans and likes to gossip with me in the lunch room. As I head up the stairs and pass John Flaxman's sculpture *St Michael Overcoming Satan*, I rearrange my face into something pleasant to hide my sadness, and go in to work.

As she grew up, Rosa's family moved between Brisbane and other properties bought and sold by her father, Thomas Murray-Prior. He was the son of an Englishman who emigrated to Sydney in 1839. While working near Maitland in New South Wales to gain experience as a pastoralist, he met the explorer Ludwig Leichhardt and travelled with him to Moreton Bay in 1843. He married Matilda Harpur in 1846 and took her back to Bromelton.

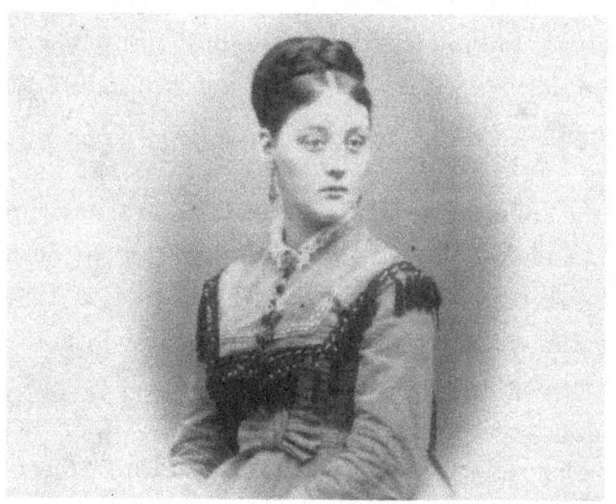

Rosa Praed, c. 1870. John Oxley Library, State Library of Queensland, Neg No: 68049

Rosa, their third child and first daughter, was educated by Matilda, who encouraged her to write. When Rosa was seventeen, Matilda died of consumption, and Rosa was so affected by the loss that her hair fell out. She took on her mother's roles: accompanying her father to Brisbane for his political business, caring for her siblings and running the house in the bush. Her marriage to Campbell Praed, the son of a lord of the manor in England, was a shock, particularly after they moved to the remote, barren

Curtis Island. By the time the Praeds sailed to London in 1876, Rosa had realised she was sexually and intellectually incompatible with her husband. Their relationship began unravelling.

In England she launched a prolific writing career that encompassed close to forty novels, thirty short stories, plays and an autobiography. In the 1880s and 1890s, her success propelled her into artistic and theosophist circles, and she counted the writer Oscar Wilde and theosophist Helena Blavatsky among her acquaintances. I'm impressed with this bush girl who grew into a canny and determined woman, using her writing to support her family and extravagant lifestyle.

One of the courses I'm taking at the London Consortium is on Stoicism, a philosophy that advocates detachment from people and things so that, if these things are taken away, it doesn't cause suffering. I'm suspicious of this. I don't see how I can stop loving Alex, or missing home so much.

I read an essay by French philosopher Michel Foucault that discusses a letter Roman emperor Marcus Aurelius wrote to Fronto, a man who was probably his lover. Marcus Aurelius was a Stoic, and in his letter to Fronto he related his day before going to bed. As Foucault describes, 'the day ends, just before sleep, with a kind of reading of the day gone by. There one unfurls in thought the roll on which the activities of the day are inscribed, and it is this imaginary book of memory that is reproduced the next day.'[8] When Fronto receives the letter, he writes to Aurelius, 'we are immediately together.'[9] In other words, reading the letter brings Aurelius's face before Fronto's, and the distance between them is annihilated.

This is why I wait fervently for emails from Alex. Whenever I read them, he's in the room with me. I write to him constantly, but his answers are few. It baffles me. I'm prepared to wait for three years until I finish my research and can go back to him. I don't countenance the thought that this might not be what he wants.

Intrigued by Rosa's first novel, I return to the British Library to start her second, *Policy and Passion: A Novel of Australian Life* (1881). It opens in a country town, a setting I know well from my childhood on a farm near Boggabri in north-west New South Wales. The description of the natural world attracts me immediately: 'A storm brooded in the distance. The oleanders and loquat-trees before the opposite houses looked brown and thirsty. The acacias in the inn garden drooped with sickly languor; and the spiky crowns of the golden pine-apples beneath them were thickly coated with dust. Flaming hibiscus flowers stared at the beholder in a hot, aggressive fashion.'[10]

Oleanders had bordered my grandmother's garden and the boundary of my primary school. We were warned not to eat them because they were poisonous. In the hills surrounding our farm, acacia burst open like stars at the end of winter. I knew, too, the sultry feeling of the air before a storm.

The novel follows the romance and fortunes of Honoria Longleat, a young Australian girl raised in the bush whose father, like Rosa's, becomes a prominent politician in Brisbane. Out on a picnic, Honoria 'rode on through tall gum-trees and yellow wattles, with here and there a clump of grass-trees, their bare stems, tufted tops, and spear-like spikes contrasting with the lank eucalypti, and breaking the monotony of foliage'.[11] As I read, I'm in the bush with her, crossing clear streams fringed with ferns, listening to the high piping of birds, the way I did when I was a girl, scrambling over limestone rocks in the bush.

The traditional owners of the land on which I was raised are the Kamilaroi people, whose country extends from Singleton in the Hunter Valley to Nindigully in south-west Queensland. I do not know the particulars of their dispossession, although from my reading of Aboriginal people's writing I have no doubt that it was dreadful. The Colonial Frontiers Massacre Map prepared by researchers at the University of Newcastle shows there was a massacre east of Manilla in 1835 by armed stockmen, and another near Barraba in 1836, and the better known 1838 Myall Creek massacre further north.[12]

In 1936, my great-grandmother Ivy Voss bought the property from the Geddes family. Before this it was part of Bayley Park, acquired by William Moore in the 1920s. Moore was a pastoralist and patron of the Wean Amateur Picnic Race Club. The picnic races are still a key social event for people in the district.

Ivy had married Frederick George White in 1905, five years after they met. George, as he was known, was working in Hughenden in north Queensland, near where Ivy lived. George was the grandson of James White, who arrived in Australia in 1826 from Somerset, England, as manager of stock for the Australian Agricultural Company. He was raised by his aunt because his mother died from complications at his birth, the doctor having been too drunk to get on his horse to attend to her. George completed an engineering degree at Cambridge in 1899, then returned to Australia where he bought a property at Richmond, some one hundred kilometres west of Hughenden. A year later, he met Ivy.

After their wedding, they moved to Sydney for a few years, then to 'Mittabah' in Exeter, New South Wales. Ivy bore twelve children between 1908 and 1930, with my grandfather arriving in 1916. After being educated by governesses, he became a weekly boarder at nearby Tudor House for two years. Patrick White, whose father was first cousin to George, attended Tudor House when my grandfather was aged five and six. On weekends, Patrick sometimes stayed with my grandfather and his family at Mittabah.

In his biography of Patrick White, David Marr writes that Patrick thought Ivy a 'monster' and kept her maiden name in mind, 'waiting for thirty years to revenge himself' with the novel *Voss*.[13] When I asked my father what Ivy was like he replied, 'She was a shit. Cold and dictating. The girls in that family were treated like slaves.'

After two years at Tudor House, my grandfather was sent to Geelong Grammar. Here, he met my grandmother, whose father was deputy headmaster of the school. He kept in touch with her when he finished his studies. After a few years of trapping rabbits on one of his father's farms, then fighting in New Guinea, my grandfather proposed to my grandmother. They married in 1942 and my grandmother lived at 'Sylvania', with Ivy and two sisters-in-law until my grandfather came back from the war, discharged with malaria and what we would now call post-traumatic stress disorder.

Ivy had purchased this piece of land among the north-west slopes and plains because, in the cold highlands of Exeter, she was homesick for the heat of her childhood home. She named it Sylvania after the property in Queensland. In summer, temperatures stretched into the forties.

After the war, my grandparents needed somewhere to live. My grandfather took out a loan from George to buy Sylvania from Ivy, but eventually his father cancelled the debt. My grandparents' three sons grew, married and brought their wives back to the farm, which, with additional purchases of nearby land, stretched to five thousand, four hundred acres. Each family had three children, bringing the number of people on the property to seventeen. The country also supported sheep and cattle, wheat, sorghum, barley, oats and, one year, a crop of sunflowers that cockatoos pecked into oblivion. Each family raised pigs, and when I was nine my father and his brothers built a much larger piggery, which they tended together. I liked to rollerskate up and down the cement aisles, as there was no other flat, hard surface on the farm.

A creek ran near our house, separating us from our grandparents' place. When it flooded, which happened every few years, Oliver and I couldn't get to school. Instead we pulled on our gumboots and stomped through boggy paddocks, damming streams and holding boat races with leaves and pieces of bark.

Dad had installed large windows in the cottage. I would sit at the table on the back verandah, drawing or doing my homework, looking out the windows. During summer storms, dark blue clouds boiled over the low hills in the distance. In the evenings, the moon rose above them, a pale disc in the indigo light.

My grandparents' house was a ten-minute walk away. It was a ten-minute run to one aunt and uncle's place, and a ten-minute drive to the other aunt and uncle's. Whenever my mother had tea with my aunts, my brother, sister and I played with our cousins. We patted horses, climbed up tankstands, dive-bombed into the pool and played hide-and-seek in an old shearing shed, which our fathers and their mates had graffitied during a wild party in the 1960s. At each child's birthday, there was an instant rent-a-crowd of Whites, who dug their fingers into bowls of jellybeans and licorice. The cake was created from the *Australian Women's Children's Birthday Cake Book*. Sometimes it was a train with licorice wheels, or a koala's face smothered in brown icing, or a pool filled with green jelly. After the party the kids sprinted around the lawn, high on sugar. We were always outside, with air, sunshine or water on our bodies. Our skin darkened in summer and lightened in winter, leaving behind a rash of freckles.

With these people, I never felt deaf. They spoke clearly and made sure they looked at me so that I could lip-read them. It helped, too, that they were all naturally loud and prone to theatrics. If I was at a social gathering, they also protected me from strangers.

At the Wean picnic races, an annual event, I wore my denim pinafore pulled over a hot-pink skivvy, Mr Men ribbons in my ponytail. I sat at the rickety folding table with Oliver and studied the photocopied race program. We selected horses based on their names and riders' colours, then traipsed after our cousins, dollar coins from Mum clasped hotly in our fists, to place bets on the horses.

At the fence surrounding the racetrack, I stood on my tiptoes, watching the small brown bunch in the distance become a mass of rippling flanks and legs, the jockeys' purple and pink silk jackets flattened by the wind. I felt the vibrations of horses' hooves in the earth as they galloped by.

'Who won?' I asked, unable to distinguish anything from the crackling voice on the loudspeaker.

'Your horse came second, Jess!'

Oliver and my cousins spoke to the bookkeeper for me. A man with a bulging belly, he stood on a wooden box, a leather satchel slung over his shoulder. He scrawled on his pad, tore it off and handed it to the boys. Oliver gave the flimsy piece of paper to me and we headed for the office, where my uncle dispensed the money, slapping a five-dollar note into my hand.

'There you go, Jessie,' he said in his gruff voice. I took the money to Mum.

'You won, darling! You can put that in your Dollarmites savings account.'

Whenever I read Rosa's novels – I'm now onto her sixth, *The Head Station* – I return to this place of lush happiness. It's a place where I was never alone and there was always sensation: static in carpets before a storm, the thick smell of flowering gum blossoms, the high-pitched yelping of farm dogs at the approach of a car, and always, in the distance, the clamour of cousins.

~

In London, it's too dark and cold to get outside much. The persistent clouds weigh me down. My weight increases, adding to my distress. I've been a runner since my teens and, although my fitness fluctuates, I'm a rat in a cage if I can't get outside. I miss the shock of my feet hitting the pavement and sweat slipping down my neck.

Uncharacteristically, because we rarely discuss our emotions, I mention my unhappiness to my mother in an email.

She replies the next day. *Migrating to country New South Wales was the hardest thing I've ever done. No one knew my background or history and it was as though I had to begin my life again.*

Mum grew up in the suburbs of Christchurch, New Zealand, helping her father in his garden on weekends. When the Beatles came to town, she stood for hours in a queue that wended around Canterbury Cathedral. She graduated from Canterbury University with an Arts degree in history and flew across the ditch to Sydney, intending to travel around the world. In Sydney she spent all her savings on frocks, so she found a job in enrolments at the Sydney Technical College. Occasionally parents tried to bribe her into enrolling their children, but she turned them away. She lived in an apartment in the harbourside suburb of Waverton, and one morning she and her flatmate planned a party. They were missing some implements, so Mum went downstairs and knocked on the door of the flat beneath hers.

My father answered it in his bell-bottoms, his shirt hanging out.

'Hi, I'm Anne. I'm from the flat upstairs. Can I borrow your fondue set? We're having a party.'

My father, James, the second of the sons, was born in 1946. Until he was twelve, he rode his bicycle for six kilometres to the bush school with his two brothers, and then home again in the afternoon. In summer they stopped to rest in the shade of trees because it was so hot. Sometimes they kicked a ball or rode their bikes over tracks made by sheep.

Their teacher lived in a tent at the back of the school and cooked his dinner on a campfire at night. The school had sixteen students and stopped at sixth grade, so at thirteen my father was sent to boarding school in Armidale with his brothers. His parents visited regularly, although it took them a whole day to make the drive.

On finishing school, Dad learned wool classing in Tamworth and worked in shearing sheds in Western Australia, saving money to go overseas. He travelled in South Africa, the Middle East, Europe and England for three years, hitchhiking and sleeping under trees. Twenty-five by the time he came home, he decided to stay in Sydney to find a wife. He wanted someone different and figured he wasn't likely to find that in the country. He picked up a job as a taxidriver, collecting passengers from the streets of Sydney in his yellow cab, while taking classes in watercolour painting at night. His mother, who did oils, had recognised his talent and encouraged him to keep painting.

Six weeks after my parents met at the door, they decided to marry. Mum's grand scheme of travelling around the world fizzled. After the wedding at Lavender Bay, at which she wore red platform shoes with her cream satin dress, they drove Dad's car, an old black Wolseley, to the farm at Boggabri. Along the way they stopped and picked up two basset hound puppies.

On the farm, Mum learned to cook on an outdoor brick stove before Dad installed a gas oven. She also began her garden, which eventually stretched into a soft lawn bordered by a rockery, roses, vegetable beds and an orchard.

I only remember Mum as happy on the farm. If she was able to settle then perhaps I will, too, if only I can work out what's going on with Alex.

The evenings draw in as Christmas approaches. Walking down Regent Street one late afternoon when it's already dark, I find lights strung across the streets in dazzling ropes of blue and red. I continue through a network of tiny lanes and end up at Trafalgar Square, where there's a group of people singing carols. I move closer to hear better. The sound is so beautiful, my heartsickness so acute, that I hurry on to fend off my tears.

On weekends, too broke to take the train, I catch a coach out of the tangled snarl of London's suburbs to visit Oliver. Because I use the cheapest company available, the coach often breaks down by the side of the road. At other times the air conditioning dies, leaving passengers gulping like fish.

Oliver is a natural performer, as are all the Whites. He relishes repeating the things I miss, adding facial expressions and actions for embellishment. When we were small, he acted out the plots of *The Cities of Gold*, *Inspector Gadget* or *Doctor Who*. Mum joked that he was my 'right-hand man' because he always stood on my right side, speaking into the ear with which I could hear.

He was born nineteen months after me and we shared the same bedroom for seventeen years. When he was small, before our sister was given her own room and Oliver slept in the trundle bed, I pulled the doona off him in the mornings to wake him up so we could play. I was never reprimanded, probably because he never complained about it to Mum. Later, he migrated to the bunk above mine. I would push my feet through the slats to poke his mattress until he laughed, or told me sharply to stop.

Aside from a year when he was at boarding school, and another four while I was at the University of Wollongong and in America, we have never lived apart. In my earliest journal, a small orange National Australia Bank notebook written over the month of May in 1988, I listed in each entry how well I had done in Maths ('I had the highest score in Maths, it was eighteen out of twenty'; 'I beat Paula G. in Maths'), then detailed the activities I did with Oliver: 'We tried to burn the dead sheep but its wool was too wet'; 'We visited the tip and I found a tennis racket and its cover and he found a hairdryer.' During Christmas holidays, saturated with heat, we dipped in and out of the pool. Underwater, we yelled at each other, our words garbled with bubbles. Surfacing and gasping, we tried to guess what the other had said. When our fingers wrinkled we climbed out of the water and sat on sun-heated flagstones outside the house. We warmed our bums and ate fat purple grapes from the vine adjacent to the cottage. Mum had tied brown paper bags around them to keep the birds out. I sent Oliver up a ladder to untie the bags and fetch me some bunches. If the cicadas were too loud, I told him to find the nearest one and stop it.

As I am unable to hear extremely high frequencies unless they are very loud, my brain is unaccustomed to processing these sounds. They always come as a shock, to the point where sirens hurt my ear and cicadas are like chainsaws. When Oliver traced the cicada to its source and stomped his foot on the ground beside it, I had a few minutes of blissful relief. Then it started up again.

There was hardly a part of the farm that Oliver and I didn't know. In the dry creek, we headed east towards its source because there was a large wire fence we couldn't scale in the other direction. On the banks, we found a rusty tap that shot out brown water when we turned it on, and old tin cans with peeling labels. Once, we came across our grandmother's dead dachshund, bloated, on the gravel floor. He'd been missing for days.

Sometimes we headed for the paddock behind our grandparents' house on the farm. Beneath a stand of pines on ground made dusty by the milking cows that rested there in the heat of the day was a square of wrought-iron fencing. The sharp, decorative palisades enclosed a small headstone, on which was written: *Hamish White, 1976 to 1977.* This was our baby brother.

'Why,' I later asked Dad as I swung on the gate to the yard at my grandparents', 'does the grave have a fence around it?'

Dad was mixing feed for some waiting calves. He placed the lid on the bucket of feed and shook it. 'To keep the cows out.'

I leaned over the gate to give it momentum. 'Why did you have it on the farm and not in town?'

Dad tipped the feed into the calves' trough. 'Town was too far away.' He didn't elaborate, and when the bucket was empty he went through the gate. I jumped off and latched it, while the calves edged towards the trough.

~

In England, Oliver and I continue our explorations. I consult the *Lonely Planet* and decide where to go, then Oliver drives us over winding roads bordered by tall hedges to National Trust homes. We amble over lawns with chiselled borders, neat gardens stretching beyond them, and listen attentively to tour guides as they lead us through dim, draughty rooms.

We also camp with Oliver's workmates on the coast at Woolacombe where there's surfing. Oliver quickly discovers that I don't like camping. The sand is grey, the waves small. I'm cold, among strangers, and haven't brought any smart clothes for dinner at the local pub, the Thatch. I sit at a long table, uncomfortable in my daggy tracksuit pants, although I'm amused when Oliver explains to his English friends the Australian connotations of 'thatch'.

To cheer me up, he drives us to a nearby town, Ilfracombe, where we find a warm café overlooking the sea. We order hot chocolates. Down at the beach, a man walks ten dachshunds beside the water, five leashes in each hand.

'Look!' I point, laughing.

The café owner brings over our mugs and says something I can't hear. Oliver repeats, 'He walks them twice a day. Once in the morning and once in the afternoon.' I laugh again, the whole damp weekend made worthwhile.

At Christmas, we head south to stay with the Blooms. Oliver worked as an au pair for their children on his gap year a few years earlier, and they 'adopted' him. Over the years in England they become my second family, too.

Our Christmases on our farm were loud and riotous, with party hats, masks, jokes and charades. One year Father Christmas pulled up in the drive of my grandparents' house in a ute, a hessian sack of presents slung over his shoulder. The kids crowded onto the lawn. I couldn't hear what he was saying, because his voice was low and I couldn't see his lips beneath the white beard. Eventually, I worked out that it was my grandfather, and I dashed forward for a present.

Being so far away from home this time, I'm glad to spend it with another large, friendly family in the country. On the Blooms' farm, we track through boggy paddocks after Nick, who's driving the tree lopper to cut down some holly.

'There's not much around,' Nick says. 'The birds have eaten most of it. I'm not sure why. It might be climate change – I've noticed the ground isn't properly cooling down over winter.'

I'm so cold I've had to buy a hideous white parka that makes me look like a walking sleeping bag. I've also asked for extra blankets to put on my bed at night.

At the end of the Blooms' driveway is a tiny church. On Christmas Eve we file in for a service with other people from their community. Although I'm an atheist, the rituals remind me of services with my grandparents at the Anglican Church in Boggabri, a solid brick building with parched lawns and a straggly gum hanging over the roof. Once again, when the carols begin my eyes burn with tears.

Afterwards, there's mulled wine in the nearby hall. The tart alcohol washes down my crumbly mince pie. This is the kind of celebration I've seen on the Christmas cards of my childhood.

The next morning when I wake up, it's snowing lightly outside. I stare out the kitchen window, dazzled.

Back in London, I come to find that January and February are the hardest months of the year. The days, which had been bearable, take on a leaden quality. The overcast sky pushes down on me and I can't keep warm. I put on more weight because shortbread is cheaper than the pleasure of buying frocks or boots.

I write to Alex, *You have been the single most important thing in my life for eighteen months and my feelings for you are so intense there doesn't seem to be words to describe them.*

The next day, a reply appears in my inbox. I open it eagerly.

Stop wasting your time on me. I don't love you.

The shortbread bubbles up into my throat, burning.

I wake in darkness. I haven't slept much but I push down the covers. No matter how much I want to stay in bed, I need endorphins to stop my depression from ballooning.

The address on Rosa's 1914 letter in Riddle's volume, which I read in the British Library, is 98 Oakwood Court in Kensington. Although a great deal of Rosa's oeuvre used Australian settings, a number of her novels are based in London, and I'm curious about her life in the city. Kensington isn't far away.

The sun is up by the time I head outside in my beanie and jumper. The dew in Hyde Park is silver and steam rises from the ponds. I stride through long, unmown grass beneath the trees. It's vaguely wild, reminding me of the bush in Australia, though it soaks my joggers and tights. I exit the park near Kensington Palace, then head to Holland Park. It's a pretty place, with wide grassy spaces and trees overhanging the paths. A handful of peacocks peck at the lawn. Their breasts are electric blue, their tails weighty with extravagance. Perhaps Rosa took her children here on sunny days.

Ninety-eight Oakwood Court is on the other side of Holland Park. It's a tall, grand set of apartments in terracotta brick. There would have been a concierge at the door who handed Rosa her letters. It would have been very different from her house in Kangaroo Point in Brisbane, a place then full of rainforest, crops and thick vegetation tumbling down to the river. London must have seemed frantic and sooty after small, quiet Brisbane.

I turn back, my breath puffing out as mist. When I get back to my room, I resolve, I'll pack my laptop and head to the British Library to read another of Rosa's novels. When that book is finished, I'll order the next one. Then I'll go to work at UCL library. When I come home, I'll keep reading. I will not think of Alex.

Still unable to sleep a few nights later, I switch the light on and read through my notes on *An Australian Heroine*. A tremor runs down my spine as I hear Esther's cry, 'Let me be free. It is all I care for. I don't want his money, or his position, or any of the fine things he has given me. I don't even want his name. Let me be myself – just Esther – free.'[14] It reminds me of Jane Eyre, climbing to the roof of Rochester's house and looking out 'afar over sequestered field and hill, and along dim sky-line', longing 'for a power of vision which might overpass that limit; which might reach the busy world, towns, regions full of life I had heard of but never seen'.[15] Jane is desperate to do what she wants, but poverty and social expectation – represented by that sweeping landscape cut up into little fields – prevent her. Just as Esther was bound by marriage. Just as I am bound by my heartsickness. We all long to pull up our skirts and run.

In my weekly class at the Institute of Contemporary Arts I start talking to the young man sitting beside me. He is always elegantly dressed.

'I'm sorry, I didn't catch your name,' I say when we rise to leave.

'It's easier if I write it down.' He writes the letters *W-o-j-t-e-k* on my notepad. 'I'm Polish,' he explains.

I also chat to a young woman, Martine, and discover that she lives in my residential college. She's a petite French Canadian from Montreal. While I walk around London in my sleeping-bag jacket, she wear singlets and cardigans.

'Aren't you cold?'

'No, this is like a Montreal spring,' she replies in her clipped accent.

At a cinema by Lancaster Gate station, we watch *2046*, the sequel to Wong Kar-wai's *In the Mood for Love*. The film centres around a philanderer, Chow Mo-wan, and his unconsummated affair with a woman. It also features lonely people trying to reach the world of 2046, where they can recapture their lost loves. It doesn't do much for my mood. I push away my thoughts of Alex and concentrate on Zhang Ziyi's elegant qípáos.

A few weeks later, Martine and I take tea in the Orangery in Hyde Park, a large-windowed building built in 1704 to protect Queen Anne's citrus trees from the winters. I like the lilt of Martine's voice and her expressive face. Her quick, clever humour makes me laugh.

I talk of my ongoing sadness about the man in Australia.

'You have given this a lot.' I hear Martine's delicate, but emphatic subtext, and file it away.

I have been in London for four months. At the end of each day, I open my desk drawer, pull out a pale yellow Post-It note and make a mark on it. In an effort stop thinking about Alex, I've forbidden myself from contacting him for two months. When I have sixty marks, I'll pick up the phone. There are still twenty-eight days to go.

I put the square back in the drawer and sit on the rough carpet on the floor. I lean my back against my bed and close my eyes.

I'm always tired; deafness absorbs a huge amount of physical energy through lip-reading, checking that I don't get run over on a road, and being constantly alert so that I don't miss someone speaking to me. My brain also has to work much harder than the average person's to process sounds with what hearing I have. But my fatigue now is abnormal; I'm utterly ground down with exhaustion. Tears seep from beneath my eyelids.

There's a flash of something sour in my mind. It makes me feel dirty, as if I don't want to be inside my head any longer. Startled, I open my eyes and wipe them with the heel of my hand. The constant crying is not right. Something in my head is not right.

At the doctor's, I blurt, 'I think I need a psychologist. I left a man behind in Australia. I can't seem to get better.' I press my fingers against my trembling lips to stop myself from crying.

The doctor touches my arm. 'You poor thing.'

I return to the clinic a few weeks later. In the psychologist's office upstairs, I find a man in his late sixties.

I talk fast with nervousness, explaining my heartache, my deafness, the eating disorder I'd had in my teens.

'Did something traumatic happen to you at puberty to make you lose weight?'

I can't think of any specific event. 'No. I just wanted to be thin.'

Within a few sessions, I become frustrated with the psychologist, who steeples his hands on his armchair and responds to my chatter with plump silences. I cancel the rest of my appointments.

An Australian friend, a well-read expatriate, tells me he went through a similar experience when he moved from Australia to London.

'I think part of the problem,' he says in his gentle way, 'is that not only have you lost Australia, but you've lost the language of Australia, too – the way you write about it. Have you thought about antidepressants?'

I shake my head. I'm petrified of feeling nothing at all. 'What if I can't write?'

~

As a writer and reader, I've learned to make patterns and links in texts. I align elements of the story according to theme and time, find resonances, and pull them together into a narrative that makes sense.

I might have a natural advantage in this process because, as a deaf person who only hears a few words, I have to form my own patterns, fitting those words together with body language, tone and facial expression into a context that creates a story. For example if, in a conversation, I hear the name of a politician such as 'Abbott' and the words 'climate change', and see a person frowning, I can surmise that they are in disagreement with Abbott's contention that coal is good for humanity.

Looking back at the conversation with the psychologist, I see that he had asked the right question and that there had indeed been trauma. Not one instance of it, but a slow and steady accretion.

~

Ruby was my best friend from age five. A photo taken by my father shows us dressed up as fairies for the Christmas play at the Mechanics' Institute building, a clapped-out piece of Art Deco architecture in Boggabri. My light-pink leotard is pulled tight over my plump tummy, from which my tulle tutu springs. Ruby's fairy frock fits her neatly. We hold our tinsel-wrapped wands, grinning at my father behind the lens.

When Ruby became a Brownie, I asked my mother if I might join Brownies as well, even though I was apprehensive about being in a hall of people I didn't know. Mum agreed and found me a Brownie uniform. She sewed a smaller version for my Cabbage Patch doll.

I became obsessed with collecting badges that I could sew onto my brown tunic, but I didn't have the social skills to carry out the activities needed to get a badge. Instead, I accompanied Ruby when she organised to have afternoon tea with an elderly lady, a friend of her family's. I sat with Ruby on the lady's verandah in a cane chair, hoping for some biscuits, unable to hear her quavering voice. For that, a badge arrived in an envelope in the post, inscribed 'Caring for Senior Citizens'. I watched with satisfaction as Mum pinned it onto my tunic and sewed it into place.

We had sleepovers at each other's houses, dragging an overnight bag to school; spent recess and lunch together, playing hopscotch or tag; and one summer we passed a week at Lake Keepit dam, a recreation park not far from Gunnedah. I enjoyed learning archery and sailing, but the sun was baking and I was surrounded by children I didn't know. When we were taken on bivouac one night, camping further along the dam, I started hyperventilating and sobbed uncontrollably. Ruby darted off and found an adult.

'What's wrong?' he asked, peering down into my face.

I hiccupped, unable to tell him that my sense of alienation was overwhelming and that I needed to be at home. The man put Ruby's arm around my shoulder and left us to it.

When Ruby's mother came to collect us at the end of the week, I collapsed in the back seat and fell asleep immediately, worn out with heat and the strain of strangers.

In my final year at primary school, I sat on a blue bench beneath the jacaranda tree in the playground. It was lunchtime. The sun was warm and a book lay open in my lap. Pale-purple blossoms were scattered at my feet, some squidged wetly into the cement. I looked up from my book to watch my classmates playing soccer on the field, shouting and calling. I would have joined them, except that of late I had felt awkward, where before I had been blithe. I, who was used to scrambling over the delightful hardness of wool bales in the shearing shed, who ran up and down the banks of creeks and crawled into tea-trees, flakes of bark sticking to my jumper, had gradually learned a consciousness of my body. *I was not like them.* Partly it was because Ruby and the girls in my year had become cliquey, clustering in tight, impenetrable groups. Although I didn't realise it then, Ruby was unsettled because her family had moved to another town, and she would soon follow them to start high school. She and I drifted apart, and at the time I couldn't understand why. My friend, once a lever, could no longer help me.

My disability support teacher, Mrs Matthews, had replaced Mr Tony when I finished Year Two. She visited once a week, checking my schoolwork, helping with my speech and talking to me about anything that was on my mind. A friendly woman who had known me for four years, she was familiar with my moods.

'Has something happened?' she asked.

I didn't have the words to articulate the sense that I was turning into something different and unlikeable, because my closest friend no longer wanted to spend time with me. Instead, I latched onto another concern. 'I'm worried that at school socials I won't be able to dance. I don't know how to do it.'

The next week Mrs Matthews brought a tape deck and we walked to the empty school hall. She plugged in the tape player.

'You know a beat, from your piano playing?'

I nodded.

'Once you have the beat, you can do anything.'

I swallowed my smile at her solid body bopping to the music. She wanted me to be happy, but instead I harboured increasing panic at the isolation that, like a cold, clammy blanket, was sticking itself onto my skin.

A few months later, the high school I would attend the next year hosted an orientation day. Mum and I sat on grass already burnt by the early summer, while a teacher described what we could expect. Nearby was a girl from my primary school. When the teacher finished speaking and we waited for another to start, the girl said, 'Hello.'

'Hi.' I plucked at the grass.

In the car on the way home, Mum castigated me, 'You were so rude to that girl! She was trying to talk to you and you didn't even reply.'

I blinked. I hadn't been aware that a conversation was necessary after someone said hello.

Children learn to socialise by listening to their family and peers, but I couldn't hear well in a group of more than two people, and had never once overheard a conversation. I had little idea of the nuance and complexity of social rules.

When I started high school, my isolation continued. I sat on the cold metal bench in the hall at lunchtime, conscious of voices echoing off the brick wall around me and fretting because I didn't know how to grab a thread and weave myself into the chatter. Time dragged. I knew instinctively not to impose on my cousin Naomi, who was in the same year as me, in case I embarrassed her. Bored and lonely, I headed to the library.

Seated at a table and soothed by air conditioning, I opened *Jodie's Journey*, a story by Colin Thiele about a girl my age with juvenile arthritis. Jodie spends her days in pain, but to all outward appearances, especially in the early stages of her disease, she doesn't look as though she has a disability.

On holidays one summer, Jodie's brother carries her down to the beach. He leaves her in the shallows while he fetches ice cream. Jodie is 'glad that the incoming ripples hid the lower part of her body and disguised the knock-kneed angle of her legs'. When a boy approaches and asks if she wants to play volleyball, Jodie has to tell him, 'I'd love to, but I can't run and jump like ordinary girls.'[16]

I knew how hard it was to say that there was something wrong with you when it didn't look like there was. I read on, engrossed.

This was the first novel I'd come across that featured a person with a disability. I was heartened by Jodie's efforts to save herself from a bushfire by tipping herself out of her wheelchair and dragging herself to the dam. People with disabilities weren't useless, but sometimes it was hard not to feel that.

I didn't encounter another novel with characters with disabilities until I was an adult, and even then they were sparse.

Halfway through the year, I sat at the table with Oliver after school, doing my maths homework. Mum joined us with a cup of tea. 'Your teacher spoke to me today. She said you spend your lunchtimes in the library.'

'I like it in the library.'

'You should try talking to people instead of reading.'

'Why?'

'Because it's good for you. Why don't you go to the oval with some friends?'

Shame welled hotly through my body. To my horror, I started to cry. 'I don't have any friends.'

Oliver and my mother stared at me. Neither of them moved, nor spoke. In the silence, I wiped my tears away, picked up my pen and continued with my equations.

~

I think about this moment as I leave my desk and walk from my apartment in East Brisbane up the hill to the bus stop. I pass grand old houses that were built when Rosa lived at Shafston House before she married, not far away at Kangaroo Point. I like looking up at them. Their verandahs and lush vegetation are similar to those in Rosa's novels.

At the top of the hill a wattle tree grows from the sandy-coloured Brisbane tuff, a type of rock formed during a volcanic explosion millions of years before. Its yellow blossoms burst open earlier each year because of our warming planet. When I see the wattle, with its tough woody stems and soft blossoms, I realise that something in me hardened after the conversation with Mum at the table. I knew I could not rely on anyone else for help and that it would be entirely up to me to resolve my problems.

I stopped spending lunchtimes in the library with characters from Libby Hathorn's *Thunderwith* and Beatrice Gormley's *Mail-Order Wings* who couldn't fit in and who escaped into the bush or sky. I sat alone on the cold metal seat in the hall adjoining the classrooms, staring at the brick wall. Chatter swirled around me. I moved my gaze to the girls nearby, who were laughing carelessly. I tried to lip-read them but I couldn't get enough of their words to work out the context. I chewed and swallowed my sandwich, the crust rasping against my throat.

When I was at primary school in Boggabri, I caught a bus from the main road with Bella and Oliver. We were the first White family on board. Another lot of cousins stepped on at the next stop and then, when we'd gone past the piggery with its sheets of aluminium shining in the morning sun, we picked up the final lot of cousins. With nine Whites aboard, the bus became noisier and noisier. One child sawed through the plastic headrest of the seat with the drawstring of her library bag, a project she'd started the week before. Two others traded jokes, laughing. Another two pored over a piece of string tangled into cat's cradle. Three of the boys played with a square of paper folded into a mouth that opened and closed. I sat on the left-hand side of the bus, so that if someone spoke to me I'd be able to hear them with the ear that had some hearing. I usually found it too hard to join in so I read my book, happy to have the noise and laughter surrounding me. When, several years later, nearly everyone left for boarding school in Armidale, I was left with this: the hollowness of a bus ride to school where their skin should have been.

Oliver went to boarding school, too, the same one my father and his brothers had attended. My mother applied to send me to the girls' boarding school in the same town, which my sister and cousins also attended, but was told I couldn't be accepted. There had been a deaf girl who'd boarded not long before, but she'd had problems with her hearing aids and wanted to go home. The school didn't want the fuss of another deaf child.

I didn't learn of this until a few years ago. When Mum told me, I burst out, 'That's totally illegal! You should have taken them to court.'

'We didn't know any different. That's just how it was.'

There were still a few cousins left on the farm. We caught the school bus to Gunnedah, but as usual I couldn't hear well enough to join in. I read my book and stared out the window at paddocks of wheat or sorghum and the shadows of trees striping the road, trying not to think about the long, empty day looming ahead.

Then I noticed him, that tall, lightly muscled boy with golden skin and large brown eyes. He was musical, good at sport, and one of the most popular boys in my year. When I stood up to get off the bus in the mornings at the school gate, my heart thudded with the anticipation of seeing him. But I was deaf and couldn't even muster a conversation with the girls I sat near at lunch, let alone a boy who made my heart thunder. I was also plump.

As a child, I was always moving. I chased the dogs around the lawn until my bare feet snapped a twig underfoot and I fell, howling. I swam furiously across a pool of muddy water at Dripping Rock to avoid leeches. In summer I tried to beat my personal best of eight laps underwater in the pool in one breath. I was good at activities that didn't need interaction with other people, but terrible at team sports because I couldn't hear where my team mates were on the field.

Meningitis had damaged my balance as well as my hearing. If I swung a bat, I usually spun around with it. I also couldn't catch because I couldn't connect a ball with my hands.

Playing cricket one evening with some cousins when I was ten, I swung the bat and missed the ball.

'I can't see it coming.'

'That's 'cause she can't see past her stomach,' added a cousin under his breath.

'What did you say?'

'Nothing.'

I was hardly overweight, but my mother sometimes said, 'You look like the side of a house.' Or, alternatively, 'like the back of a bus'.

Food was abundant on the farm. Oliver and I climbed over the fence to the orchard, lifting up netting that protected the trees from fruit bats, and pulled off nectarines, peaches, oranges and mandarins. For twenty cents from Mum we'd gather an ice-cream container full of strawberries from the patch, popping one in our mouths and another into the container. The strawberries burst, hot and sweet, in our mouths.

Mum barely knew how to cook when she married, but she learned to make roasts and quiches, trifles, pecan pie, pear flans and chocolate mousse. On holidays and weekends we ate our main meal in the middle of the day, because Dad needed energy to labour on the farm. We sat on the enclosed verandah that looked out to the hills, eating lamb chops, mashed potato and broccoli draped in a béchamel sauce flavoured with cheese. I didn't want the fatty rind on my chop because it was overpowering, so I gave it to Mum.

'Don't eat that,' my father said to her. 'You'll get fat.'

'Be quiet.'

Oliver wiped his plate clean with a finger and sucked it.

'Use your fork,' Mum told him. 'And Jess, bring the dessert bowls please.'

I counted five bowls from the cupboard and five spoons from the dresser and brought them to the table. Bella was prattling about school. I couldn't tell if anyone was listening.

Mum followed me with a dish fresh from the oven, wrapped in a tea towel to keep her hands from burning. She laid it in the centre of the table on a placemat.

'Chocolate self-saucing pud!' Oliver announced.

Mum ladled the pudding and sauce into bowls and passed around a jug of cream. When it reached her, she tipped a thin stream into her pudding. Dad said, 'You can't have that, you'll get fat.'

She ignored him and wiped drips from the lip of the jug with her spoon.

Perhaps my father was joking when he made these references. Maybe he and my mother shared a language in which these comments were code for something affectionate. To me, though, it sounded like criticism.

My sister Bella, now a mother, has a daughter who is a teenager. I've exhorted her never to mention her daughter's weight, explaining the conversations I'd heard at the dinner table.

'I have no recollection of them whatsoever,' Bella replies.

It must have been a difference in our perspectives. Ever confident, Bella sailed through adolescence, whereas I, who watched and listened to everything that was unsaid, learned this: that a woman could not be acceptable, nor even lovable, unless she was thin.

Mum was often trying diets or going on health retreats with her Sydney friend, the one with whom we'd stayed when I went to the audiologist to be diagnosed.

'I'm going to start walking around the paddocks for exercise, Jess,' she announced.

I thought of the golden-skinned boy who, I had no doubt, wouldn't look at me unless I was thinner. 'I'll come with you.'

After a few weeks of walking, we worked up to a jog. Mum lost interest, but I kept going.

When I came home from school, I exchanged my black lace-ups for sneakers and ran into the paddocks. The wind flattened my T-shirt against my belly, spinifex scratched my shins and burrs furred my socks. I scarcely saw the clumps of dirt and rock on the ground before me, I could only see the boy waiting at the wire fence that marked the paddock's boundary. My knees hurt and my breath was ragged, but I wouldn't stop. I sprinted until I reached the fence, sagging onto it with relief. With another breath, I climbed the fence and kept going, even though it was like running on knives.

I ran for half an hour every afternoon, with Saturday off, and for an hour on Sundays. I ran through the hills at the back of our house, my joggers slipping on bark and leaf litter. Heat rose from the earth and coiled around my ankles. At my footfall, roos bounded away and wild goats stepped nervously through pine trees. On hot summer days, I defied my mother and ran in the baking heat. Clouds of locusts lifted from the dry grass as my feet slammed down. Up in the hills, slabs of granite gave off a warm, clean scent and cicadas wove a thicket of sound.

In winter, I ran as the sun went down. Dew drew out the rich smell of soil, while cooling air tightened the sweat on my skin. In spring, the gum blossoms thickened the air with sweetness and wattle burst from the palette of olive and grey trees.

The solitude was a balm. There were no conversations to tax me, no one to please, no anxiety from failing to respond or act in the correct way. The only expectation was to put one foot in front of another and to make sure I didn't step on snakes. I came close to it, startling one near my foot as I daydreamed about the boy's hand on the back of my neck. The snake looped away over the fence.

Whenever I read Rosa's novels, I reconnect with this heady mix of romance and the bush. In *Policy and Passion*, the foil of Honoria, the headstrong protagonist, is Angela, a sickly slip of a girl who is obsessed with art. Barrington, an Englishman, comes across her in the bush:

> It was a pretty, secluded spot. The creek-sides rose high and shelving, and were overgrown with mulgam plants now past fruiting, ferns, and a stiff green grass, of which the yellow bloom emitted a powerful aromatic perfume.

> As Barrington let his horse drink, his eyes wandered aimlessly along the banks, and a little distance down the stream were attracted by the flutter of a white dress through the trees.
>
> A girl poised lightly upon a slippery log, which spanned a pool deep enough to render the prospect of immersion sufficiently alarming. She appeared to hesitate whether or not to advance, nervously drawing back her foot and clutching at the swaying branches of a wattle-tree that overhung the narrow bridge.[17]

As I read this, I'm a girl on the bus again, travelling between home and school, watching cockatoos flash through the trees, thinking about the boy I'll see that day, imagining him holding my hand or carrying my schoolbag heavy with books.

Beyond the bus's rattling windows are grey–green gums, pine trees and low granite outcrops dotted with prickly pear, all interspersed with paddocks crammed with rust-coloured sorghum. Closer to town, where there's access to the river for irrigation, there are crops of cotton, white boules cracking open from brown stems. I imagine walking with the boy through the long, pale wiregrass, then lying next to him on a sun-warmed slab of granite encrusted with lichen.

Perhaps, in London, Rosa escaped to the bush in her mind as a way of finding succour, the way she physically plunged into the bush as a girl, as I did when I came home from school. Nearly half of her output features scenes from her early childhood. Even after her novels about feminism and the occult became popular, she continued to source details about Australia, usually from her correspondents. She described this as 'copy' and included it in her novels.[18] Writing about Australia and writing to people in Australia was a way of bringing them close. For both her and me, the bush helped to restore our selves.

Even as I found a salve through running, I was permanently tired, my knees hurt and I would rather have lain on my bed, reading. But if I didn't run, my hatred of myself would have been unbearable.

As I trudged along the gravel road back to our house one afternoon, my grandfather pulled up beside me in his ute.

'Do you want a lift, Jess?'

I shook my head. 'I'll be right.'

'You sure?'

'Yes, thanks.'

He drove away slowly so as not to bathe me in dust. He didn't understand that the point of running was to run, not to be driven.

I no longer ate biscuits at morning tea or dessert after dinner. When an aunt picked me and her daughters up after school and stopped at the local fryer for hot chips, I refused every chip that was offered to me, even though I adored their crispness and the way my tongue curled at the touch of chicken salt.

'Are you sure you don't want any, Jess?' my cousins asked.

'Yes.'

On another occasion, I met Mum at the other aunt's house, after I'd run the seven kilometres between us. This aunt's kitchen was dark blue and yellow; whenever I smell nutmeg, now, I'm reminded of it. My aunt made a pot of tea for us and set it down on the table with a plate of apricot slice.

'Would you like some, Jess?'

'No, thank you.'

My aunt turned the pot and poured the tea, chatting to my mother. After a while, she broke off and turned to me. 'Just try a piece, Jess. It doesn't have anything bad in it, just apricot, oats, coconut and some butter and sugar.'

Not wanting to be rude, I picked up a piece and nibbled the corner. The sharp, sweet apricot burst in my mouth and coconut brushed over my tongue. I ate the rest of the slice in silence.

Although I didn't let myself eat much, I became fixated on recipes. I looked up *julienne* in the dictionary and applied it to a pile of carrots. I could make a chocolate cake from memory. I boiled rice in chicken stock and carefully closed the sticky grains around cubes of cheese to make arancini balls. Making sure other people had food, and that I didn't, meant victory.

As I cooked and ran, bruises clustered on my skin from vitamin deficiencies. One, on the smooth skin inside my arm, was the green–blue colour of clouds before a hailstorm. My periods, which had just started, stopped for two years. I became so thin that I couldn't keep warm. In winter I shivered constantly in the school's cold, catholic rooms. Once, I saw the boy I adored at a desk across the aisle, laughing with the girl next to him, shaking his body. Unreasonably, I assumed they were laughing at my own body's constant shaking to warm itself. That evening, I asked my mother to buy me a parka.

Every afternoon I fell asleep on the bus home from school. On weekends, I lay on the bed in my father's studio, listening to music, too exhausted to move. Sometimes, when I had more energy, I bashed the piano keys in fury and slammed doors so hard that the glass rattled. I often shouted at my parents. I had no friends and I missed my brother. I was obliterated by loneliness.

Even as I was destroying my body, I began to have conversations with the girls who sat next to me at lunch. Running and starving gave me confidence, for I was in command of my body when everything else was beyond my control. Although the only thing I knew how to talk about was assignments and schoolwork, the girls I sat with didn't seem to mind.

After a parent–teacher evening, my mother said, 'The teachers have noticed that you're doing better. You're talking to people. That's really good, Jess.'

I brightened. This was an improvement on the last parent–teacher evening in which, when my teachers had reported on my compliance and discipline, my father replied, 'She's terrible when she gets home. She slams doors and shouts at us.'

A few months ago, as I scrawled this account in the sticky Brisbane heat, my neighbour's grey cat Pierre sprawled over the papers on my table, I pulled my laptop towards me and emailed my parents, *What was it like to have a deaf child?*

My father replied, *I couldn't understand why you were so bad-tempered, and now I realise it was because you were frustrated.* Yet I recall an earlier conversation I'd had with him in my twenties in which he'd said, 'We know Jessica is finding it difficult, we'll just let her slam the doors.' Perhaps this is any parent's attitude to their teenager.

It never occurred to him or my mother to counsel me or to find out what the underlying problems were. To them, I was just an exceptionally trying adolescent, so they didn't look further afield for answers. I couldn't address the situation either. After the conversation at the table with Oliver and my mother, I sensed that I couldn't trust them, or anyone else, to help me, even if I was able to find the words to express what was happening to me. I was locked into myself, battling to survive.

I try to think what could have helped when I was young. A good school counsellor, certainly. A deaf friend, who would have made me feel less strange and alone. An environment in which I could have communicated my emotions, rather than bottling them up.

It's easy to make these kind of observations in retrospect. It's also easy to see, which I couldn't possibly have done at the time, that by enduring my excruciating loneliness, I found a reservoir of strength and resourcefulness. I learned resilience and worked out problems without asking for help, which meant I developed skills in lateral thinking. I focused unreservedly on my schoolwork because this was an area in which I excelled and that made me feel better about myself. This, in turn, gave me a pathway to a career in writing and academia.

Each of these qualities turned me into a woman who could fix her mind upon a goal and work, regardless of hardship, until she achieved it. All of the things one needs, in fact, to survive as a writer.

Once again, deafness was a *pharmakon*, both poison and cure.

Looking at the bruises and my angular hipbones as I stood on the scales each night, Mum concluded that my refusal to eat was not some passing diet, and spoke to the family doctor. When she picked me up from the bus one afternoon, there was a Mars Bar sitting behind the gearstick.

'You don't have to eat all of it. Just try some. The doctor says your stomach has shrunk so much you feel full as soon as you eat something, so we have to make it bigger again.'

I stared at the Mars Bar, debating with myself. Then, ever obedient, I reached for it, unpeeled the wrapper and carefully bit into it. The chocolate was so sweet it hurt.

'Never use the word "pain",' I tell my creative writing students at the university in Brisbane. 'It's too abstract for readers to conceptualise. Instead, you need to pin concrete images to the emotion to help them to see it.'

Pain was sitting on the bus reading because I didn't have enough hearing to join in on the conversations of my cousins, baffled by how they could chat and laugh so easily. It was looking up from my book at sunlight splintering through the gum trees, blinding me with its loveliness. It was asking, through one of the girls I had come to know, if the golden-skinned boy would go out with me. The answer came back with a laugh, more nervous than unkind.

'He said no.'

I was careful to hold my expression steady.

A year after this, we moved off the farm to Armidale, where Dad began a job as an art teacher. I became a daygirl at the boarding school that had previously rejected me, which now had a new principal, a tall, graceful woman who was aware of my deafness and took care to make sure I could hear.

I felt safer in this place, despite a ritual of abuse on the way to school. In the mornings, I made a much shorter trip on the bus than on the farm, but I was always late because the bus went to the state high school first. My principal contacted the bus company and asked if they could drop me off first and then go to the high school, which began classes later.

I was the only private-school girl on the bus and the kids from the high school jeered at me as soon as the route changed. I couldn't hear their words, only that there was a large volume of noise coming from the back of the bus.

A couple of times the driver, who was a woman, stopped the bus and said, 'Leave the girl alone!'

As she drove on, the kids started up again. I turned my hearing aid off and stolidly read my book. If they were so stupid that they wanted to abuse a deaf girl, I decided, that was their problem. I always took care to thank the driver when I stepped off at school.

One morning the back tyre of the bus banged like a gunshot.

'I've never had a blowout before!' said the driver, shaken. She called the headquarters on her radio. We filed off and waited for someone to come and help change the tyre. Some kids dawdled by the side of the road, or leaned against the wire fence of a nearby garden. A rosebush from the garden spilled over the fence. I moved away and steadfastly ignored everyone in case they harassed me. When we traipsed back onto the bus, I found a rosebud on my seat. A boy must have picked it from the garden as we waited.

The world, I was learning, was full of people both kind and unkind.

Meanwhile at school, if the girls bitched, I never heard them. I made cautious friendships, which slowly strengthened. Oliver became a day pupil at the boys' boarding school and lived at home. We weren't as at ease with one another as we had been on the farm, but I was more secure with him around. The town was tranquil, although I disliked the monotony of houses and running on hard, sealed roads. We were given hearty lunches at school. I exercised less fervently and felt less anxious. I began to gain weight again.

When I look back on this period, now, I can see that the elderly psychologist, for all his reticence, had asked the right question. In London, the old trauma of being separated from all that had kept me moored – the bush, my family, my lover – had resurfaced. I was at sea, and the water was cold and bitter.

~

From the drawer of my desk in my tiny room in the college in London, I take out the yellow Post-It note. It's now filled with twelve bunches of crossed-out marks. I sit on my floor, pull the phone towards me and dial Alex's number. My heart beats in my throat as I wait for him to pick up. The tension is made worse by the fact that I dislike communicating by phone, except with my family, because I can't see people's faces to read their lips and expressions.

'Hello?'

'Hi, it's Jess.'

'Hi.'

'How are you?'

'Not bad.'

'I thought I'd ring and see how you are.'

'I'm fine.' His tone is terse.

Falsely bright with panic, I tell him about my research. He doesn't respond. After a few more awkward minutes of stilted conversation, I hang up.

Later, he emails, *You didn't write to me for two months. I don't see why I should have been welcoming.*

I re-send the email I'd written two months before, explaining why I needed to stop writing to him. Apparently he hadn't received it. I don't see why that mattered.

I tear up the Post-It note into crumbs of yellow paper and flush them down the toilet.

I walk to Edgware Road in the next suburb for groceries. There's surprisingly little traffic and I'm confused for a moment, wondering if it is in fact Sunday, not a weekday. Outside Edgware Road Station there's police tape. Perhaps there's been a car crash nearby.

I buy my groceries and return to Talbot Square. My mobile, which I'd left behind on my desk, shows two missed calls from Oliver. A text is waiting for me too. *Jess, you alive? There have been bomb attacks in London, three of them on public transport. Message me back asap. Love Oliver.*

I'm fine, I text.

I wonder whether to go into work. Unaccustomed to using the phone, it doesn't occur to me to call my boss and ask her. I don't know what else to do. I pack my satchel and head out.

London is usually crammed with people and cars, but the streets are empty except for a few black cabs. At work, my boss greets me with amazement. 'What are you doing here? Didn't you hear what's happened?'

'I wasn't sure if work was on, so I decided to come in.'

'A bomb went off at Tavistock Square, two blocks away! We're shutting the library down.'

With my colleagues, I cluster at the window to try to see what's happening at Tavistock Square, but I'm too short. After a while, my colleagues disperse and I shoulder my satchel again.

Only when I head back do I begin to be frightened. The streets, now even emptier, are silent and eerie. Police direct people as they try to find a way out of the area that's been locked down. I join trails of people walking out of the city like ants, and realise I should have checked the news before I headed out.

When I get back to my room, I text Martine, who has moved out of the residential college to a place in East London. *Are you okay, love?*

I walked home in high heels. It took me two hours.

You poor thing. Glad that you're safe.

A biography I've ordered, *Rosa! Rosa!*, arrives in the mail. It's by Patricia Clarke, a historian and writer who has published on colonial women writers. As I begin to read it I realise, with a rush of excitement, that one of the houses in which Rosa lived is in the same square as the concrete bunker of my residential college, at number 16. In addition, Praed Street, the main street of Paddington where I disembark from the bus, was named after her husband's ancestor William Praed.

It was through the Praed family that Rosa was at last able to realise her ambition of becoming a writer. In her childhood, with her mother's encouragement, she had been the main contributor to the family's handwritten monthly periodical, the 'Maroon Magazine'.[19] When she grew older and her father bought Shafston House in Brisbane, she sat on the verandah discussing her future with her friends, and declared she intended to be an author.[20] From Curtis Island, where she moved with Campbell, Rosa sent stories to editors in Sydney, but they weren't successful. In England she continued to write, even when her manuscripts were regularly returned from publishers.[21]

Campbell, having proven a poor property manager on Curtis Island, had taken over the running of a brewery back in England at Wellingborough, which he'd bought in partnership with his brother and cousin.[22] He moved the family to Rushden, next to Rushden Hall where the Sartoris family lived. Frederick Sartoris was an author, and he became a mentor to Rosa, encouraging her to achieve her literary aspirations. Through Campbell's brothers Rosa met Frederic Chapman, one half of the publishing duo Chapman and Hall, who also published Charles Dickens, William Makepeace Thackeray, Thomas Carlyle and George Meredith. The latter was one of the initial readers of the manuscript that would become Rosa's first novel, *An Australian Heroine*. His criticism was harsh, but after at least a year of hard work and rewriting, her novel made its way into print.[23]

I feel the frisson of connection, identifying with Rosa's repeated rejections, the audacity of beginning and persisting with a novel, and her move to London, which opened up her world. Just as I have Patrick White lingering in my literary history, so too did Rosa have poets in her background: her mother's father, Thomas Harpur; her stepmother's mother, Emily Barton; and her stepmother's nephew, Banjo Paterson.[24]

And, like Rosa, I find my feet as a writer in London.

Before I left for England, I quit my dreary job of writing letters about parking fines and returned to Armidale, where I house-sat for my parents while they travelled. I worked on the manuscript for my first novel, trying to fix the voice, which didn't seem to be working. With the help of a mentorship from the Australian Society of Authors, which paid for an editor, I set about rewriting it. When the draft was finished, I found an agent and packed my bags for London. Consumed with the stress of relocating, I largely forgot about the book.

One morning a few months after the bombing I wake up, check my emails and gasp: my agent has written to say that Penguin has offered to publish *A Curious Intimacy*. I scramble up and do three star jumps, then pick up the phone to call my mother.

'Well done, dear. That's wonderful.' When I put the phone down, I'm buzzing. After lunch I belt into work, shouting, 'Guess what?' My colleagues look up, their faces lightening at my rush of energy. 'I'm going to be an author! Penguin is going to publish my book!'

To celebrate, I organise drinks on the rooftop of the Castle, a pub in Angel at which I often drink with Martine and Wojtek. The sun generously makes an appearance.

A room in Martine's house becomes available. It's more affordable than the residential college, so I catch a bus to East London to check it out. I travel past a part of the city I've never visited before: the Barbican, an arts centre built in the ruins of the Second World War; the bright clutter of Smithfield Markets; a city farm strewn with straw, where I disembark. Goats nuzzle grass at the fence as I pass.

The townhouse is part of a block of housing commission apartments beside Regent's Canal. Its carpet is a lurid swirl of brown and yellow, and the cream-coloured wallpaper is textured. The third flatmate, also studying at the London Consortium, is Australian. On the walls hang his small, square canvases of horses and riders tumbling through the air.

Although the place is nowhere near as close to work or my classes as the college, the room is cheap and I enjoy Martine's company. I decide to move in.

I still walk everywhere as I've gone up a dress size, but my step is lighter. It takes an hour to get to work from my new home, following the path beside Regent's Canal. As the days warm, I do away with my possum-fur gloves and beanie, gifts from my grandmother in New Zealand, but I still need the hideous parka.

I look out for cyclists whizzing along, as I can't hear them coming up behind me. If it's sunny, I can watch for their shadows on the pavement, but otherwise it's a case of keeping as far to the left as I can. I emerge at Angel and weave through streets lined with elegant terrace houses, admiring bare trees beginning to fizz with blossoms.

One Friday evening after work, I buy a bottle of milk from the supermarket on Broadway Market and walk down Pownall Road to our townhouse. Martine and Wojtek are at a housewarming party of mutual friends, but it's the end of a week of work and listening and I'm too tired to go along.

As I walk I daydream, a habit left over from the farm when I dawdled along levee banks, dragging a stick behind me to feel the satisfying vibrations of it rattling in the dirt. I think of Coogee Beach in Sydney, to which Oliver and I often caught the bus when summer's heat sapped us. I sense someone behind me and glance around. There's a man a few paces back. I look across the road. A girl is walking on ahead. Nothing seems out of the ordinary. I turn left into the paved area between our block of flats and the road. A few cars and the recycling and garbage bins are parked here. Beyond them, two men unload a van. There's a covered way between this area and the grassy space surrounded by the flats. The man follows me but I don't think anything of it.

When I pass under the covered way his arms close around me. Adrenalin floods my body, the way it does when I wake from a nightmare. I roar. The man puts his hand over my mouth. His little finger catches between my teeth and I bite down hard. His grip loosens and I twist out of his arms. He lets go and walks away.

I stare after him, trying to get an image that I can describe to the police, but all I can see is that he's tall. I remember the pinkness of his palm as his hand closed over my mouth. His smell, of something unwashed, is on my skin and his blood is in my mouth. As soon as I unlock my door I run to the kitchen sink and spit it out.

I dial emergency services. They say they'll send the police around. I'm desperate to have a shower to get the man's smell off my skin but I can't risk not hearing the police arrive.

It takes an hour for the police to turn up.

'Sorry we're late,' the two men say. 'We couldn't find your apartment. We've looked for CCTV footage but the camera didn't reach under that covered way. Can you tell us what happened?'

I describe the attack. One policeman writes in his notebook.

'Did the man say anything to you?'

'I'm pretty deaf, so he might have, but I don't think so. I would definitely have heard him if he was shouting.'

'Did he try to grab your bag?'

'No. His grip was soft. The only unusual thing I can remember was that his hands smelled sour, like they hadn't been washed for a while. What about AIDS?'

'Did you draw blood?'

'Yes. I spat it in the sink. Sorry, I guess you could have used the DNA.'

'Have you got any cuts in your mouth?'

I shook my head.

'It's unlikely. The blood goes down your throat and into your digestive system. If there's a cut, that's how it gets into your bloodstream. But get a test, anyway.'

'Okay.'

'Have you got someone you can be with? It's better not to be on your own.'

'My flatmate's at a party.'

'Where is it? We might be able to take you there.'

'Wood Green, I think.'

They shake their heads. 'That's too far away for us. Give her a call and see if she can come home.'

'Okay.'

When the policemen leave, I take a long shower, then I phone Oliver.

'Hi Jess, what's up?'

I hesitate.

'What's the matter?'

'I got attacked by a man who followed me home.'

'Jesus Christ!'

I call Martine, who suggests I catch a taxi to where the party is. Numb, I do as she says. When I reach the door of the house, she and Wojtek hug me. They find me a drink and I distract myself by talking to people. I'm wearing a new perfume by Nina Ricci. I'm never able to use it again.

It wasn't the actual attack that upset me most. The reason I came to loathe London so much lay in the two men unloading a van, four metres away, who would have heard me scream but didn't come to help. Nor did anyone in the surrounding flats open their doors.

It's a commonly cited statistic that one in three women experience sexual or physical violence at some point in their lives. I don't know if my deafness made me more vulnerable than a hearing person. Although I knew the man was behind me, I hadn't been able to hear how close he was, nor the rustle of fabric as he lifted his arms to grab me.

I ask a friend who has all his hearing, 'If someone was walking behind you, would you be able to hear them?'

'Yeah, though probably not if I was drunk.'

Even now, ten years after the attack, if I walk through the sunlit streets of Brisbane and someone appears without warning at my side, my heart contracts.

Two weeks after the assault, I sign up for a self-defence course. Oliver offers to pay for it because I'm so broke.

'Girls are taught not to fight back,' says the instructor. 'They think that if they're passive and do what the guy wants, it won't be as bad. But that's not right. If you fight back, it can be scary for the guy. Women fight differently to men. They use teeth and nails and go for vulnerable places. That gives men a fright. They're going to stop and wonder if you're really worth the struggle.'

The attack on me was over in one minute and I had acted purely on instinct. I put it down to years of fighting with Oliver when we were children. I'd wrestle and tickle him until he was flat on the floor, then sit on his back until he couldn't breathe from laughing.

A few months later, Oliver tells me of a dream he'd had. 'There were some men who were after you, and you couldn't hear them coming. They were going to catch you and do bad things to you.'

I start to detest the area I live in. I rarely stay out late and resent the darkness of the long evenings; they leave me blind as well as deaf, and I feel even more vulnerable. I wait impatiently for the days to bloom further into spring, but that's a while away. It's so cold that Regent's Canal has frozen over. I stop before it on my way to work, admiring the way the morning sunlight reflects the sheets of ice, my fear momentarily forgotten.

Just as I had thought I was coming to like London, my unhappiness resurges. I correct my habit of daydreaming and glance often over my shoulder, checking to see who is behind me.

~

Sometimes I meet people in Brisbane's bars and tell them my history, the way you do when you're creating a self for strangers. Their faces light up when I mention the years I spent in London.

'That must have been fantastic!'

'It wasn't.'

When I explain my homesickness, the lack of sunlight, the man I left behind, the bombs and the physical assault, their brows furrow.

'Why didn't you go home?'

'I had a scholarship and I didn't want to give it up.'

This is the simple answer. The complicated answer is that it never occurred to me to leave. Writing and academic achievement were compensation for years of loneliness and social awkwardness at school and university. If I gave them up, I'd have nothing.

There was also something else. A discovery. From Clarke's biography, I learned that Rosa's first child, born in 1874, was a girl named Matilda Elizabeth, or Maud. Her pet name was 'the Bird of Paradise' or 'Birdie'. When she was two years old, just before the Praed family set sail for England, it was discovered that she couldn't hear.

This girl, I come to learn over the next decade, is a key to unlocking my understanding of my deafness and of myself.

It isn't clear how Maud became deaf. Rosa didn't think she had been so at birth, remarking in a letter to her stepmother that Maud 'was nervous because she started at the slam of a door' (although, I think, it could also have been the vibrations of the slam that startled her).[25] It was only when an uncle rang a bell behind Maud's head, not long before they set sail for London, that Rosa realised her daughter was deaf. She thought that Maud might have lost her hearing when they were living on Curtis Island. Rosa had noticed an unpleasant smell coming from Maud's ears, but instead of taking the baby, then four months old, to a doctor across the strait to the mainland (which would have been difficult regardless), she syringed Maud's ears.[26]

When I describe this to a friend with a nursing background, she winces. 'If the baby's ears were so infected that they smelled, you wouldn't go sticking anything into them!'

Although Rosa had access to her father's library and was a knowledgeable observer of his involvement in politics, her education wouldn't have prepared her for raising a deaf child. She described Maud's condition to her stepmother Nora as 'a sore heartbreak to me', and her first thoughts on arranging Maud's future were, 'if it should be that she was born deaf we must have her taught at Home'.[27] She resolved that 'as soon as we get to London we shall take her to a good aurist and learn the truth'.[28] In a letter written when she was thirty, Maud referred to 'Dr Cumberbatch, the eminent oral surgeon'. This was Alfonso Elkin Cumberbatch, the first Aural Surgeon of St Bartholomew's Hospital in London. Maud's mention of him suggests that, at some point, Rosa had Maud examined in the hope of a cure.[29]

It eventually became apparent to Rosa that Maud's hearing loss was permanent. In 1880, four years after their arrival in England, she decided against home tutoring and enrolled her six-year-old daughter in a school in Ealing, London, run by a teacher training college, the Society for Training Teachers of the Deaf and the Diffusion of the 'German' System. This school was established in 1878 by a British Member of Parliament, Benjamin St John Ackers, whose only child was deaf. Ackers and his wife had sent a teacher, Arthur Kinsey, to Europe and the United States to learn the 'German', or oral method, which taught deaf children to speak. The opposite system was the 'French' system, which taught deaf people to communicate using sign language, a far easier method.

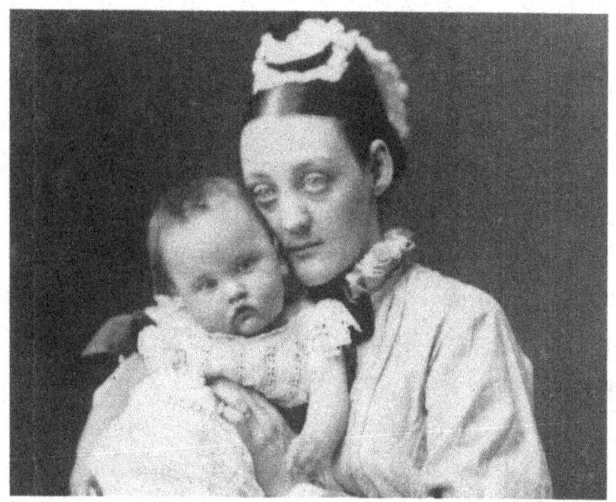

Rosa with Maud at age ten months. John Oxley Library, State Library of Queensland, Neg No:197580

~

My parents had little experience of deaf people, and none of deaf children. At the forefront of their minds was the question, as it is with any parent, of how they could arrange the best possible life for me, given that they lived on a property in rural Australia that was a long way from services.

I email Mum to find out what it was like for her when she discovered I was deaf. She replies, *At the time of finding out there was huge fear, lack of understanding and no one to turn to. We have never ever, even now met another deaf person or parents thereof.*

This is not quite true. There was a family in Gunnedah with whom we'd had afternoon tea when I was in secondary school. Their toddler was deaf and they, too, had been overwhelmed. Some ten years later we ran into the family on a street in Kensington, Sydney. The girl had a cochlear implant and was doing well at school.

I email Mum again. *Why didn't you seek out other deaf families?*

She replies, *We have to plead ignorance on all fronts. There was nothing in the country to offer assistance. I guess we just subconsciously decided to do what we could for you within the family and the school.*

These days the internet is a godsend for people who need to find out about deafness, but when my parents moved to the farm in 1972, they only had one telephone line, known as a party line, for all the properties in their area. They needed to dial the telephone exchange in Boggabri using a Morse code of long and short rings, then their call was placed through. They could only work out if someone was calling them by listening to the pattern of rings. With such antiquated technology, it's no wonder it was hard for them to meet the parents of other deaf children. Besides, to all appearances, I was doing well and was happy with my siblings and cousins on the farm. My parents' priority was to ensure, as with my brother and sister, that I achieved well academically.

When I recovered from meningitis, Mum bought a packet of large, brightly coloured letters and kept them under the antique dresser in a long, grey cardboard box. I was so enamoured of those pink, green, red and yellow shapes that the dresser gave off a delicious aura.

'Mum,' I asked, dragging the box out as my mother made lunch, 'can I do my words?'

'In a moment. When I've put the carrots on.'

While the carrots simmered, Mum sat on the rough camel-hair carpet beside me and lifted out the shiny sheaves of letters, forming them into words. Watching me, she figured I would cope at the local primary school with my siblings and cousins. It was a small school where I wouldn't be overwhelmed. At the most its combined population from Kindergarten to Year Six was one hundred and ten pupils. The government, my parents also found, provided funding for a teacher for the deaf to visit and help with my speech and schoolwork.

Sometimes Mum and Dad discussed sending me to the Shepherd Centre, a school for deaf children in Sydney, but it was a six-hour drive away and I was too young to board. It was also too difficult for my father to leave the land and move us to the city.

Mum and I did make a trip to Sydney, though, to meet a woman who ran an organisation for deaf people. Libby Harricks was a friend of the couple with whom Dad and I had stayed the first time we went to the hearing specialist. Libby became deaf when she had small children, and committed herself to raising awareness about deafness. She was a founding member and long-term president of SHHH Australia (Self-Help for Hard of Hearing People), and represented the needs of deaf and hearing-impaired people on the Sydney 2000 Olympics Access Committee. Later, she was made a Member of the Order of Australia in recognition of her efforts for deaf and hearing-impaired people. Sadly, she died of cancer at age fifty-two. Mum and Dad's friend, who had introduced us to Libby, also died of cancer around this age.

I was six when Mum drove us to Libby's office in Pymble in north Sydney. I sat on a chair, too short for my feet to touch the floor, and swung my legs. I was bored because I couldn't hear the conversation, but I knew this woman was important in some way and that she, like me, was deaf.

I realise now that the visit was more for Mum than me. Libby reassured Mum that she was on the right track with sending me to a mainstream school, particularly as there weren't any other practical options available. Besides, as I was bright and learned fast, there didn't seem to be any other problems for them to work on aside from my speech and social awkwardness.

We just got on with life and you fitted in as best you could, Mum explained.

I don't begrudge the choice my parents made in sending me to a mainstream school because this ultimately led me to books and writing, my raison d'être. Yet I was alarmed, as I researched the history of the deaf to contextualise Maud's experiences, to find that the desire to mainstream deaf children had a long and sinister history.

Signing is a natural tendency for humans. There is Palaeolithic evidence that visual-based languages came before auditory language, and sign language was in use from at least the fifth century BCE. A Greek vase dated from this time shows Philomela, whose tongue was cut out by King Tereus of Thrace, using signs. A year later, in Plato's *Cratylus*, Socrates asks, 'if we had no faculty of speech, how should we communicate with one another? Should we not use signs, like the deaf and dumb? The elevation of the hands would mean lightness, heaviness would be expressed by letting them drop.'[30]

Despite this early evidence of communicating through sign, it was thought that deaf people couldn't be educated and that they were more like animals than people. This was because speech was associated with reason. In the Enlightenment, the voice was the vessel of reason and reason was the essence of being human. St Augustine (354–430) had claimed that 'Faith comes from hearing', and if deaf people couldn't hear the word of God, they couldn't be Christian.[31] Further back still, in ancient Roman law, deaf people were placed in the same category as imbeciles.

These ideas persisted for nearly two thousand years, until monks such as Fray Pedro Ponce de León (1520–84), who educated the deaf children of aristocratic Spanish families in the sixteenth century, proved that deaf people could be taught to speak. The aristocrats were anxious to pass on their wealth and wanted to make sure that their children were educated and seen as people before the law. As Harlan Lane writes in *When the Mind Hears*, 'a mute was not a person at law', so communication was necessary to prove personhood.[32]

Sign language was used in religious communities, such as de León's Benedictine Monastery of San Salvador at Oña in Burgos, Spain, which had taken a vow of silence. Two of de León's deaf charges, brothers Francisco and Pedro de Velasco, came from a family of four deaf children. They would have devised their own system for signing within their family because children who are deaf but whose parents do not sign generally develop their own system of gestures, known as 'home sign' or 'kitchen sign'. If there is more than one deaf child in the family, this system develops into a more sophisticated private language.

The de Velasco boys would have been grateful for each other's company as they travelled through rocky slopes, gorges and forests of beech, oak, pine and juniper on the journey to the monastery. Once they arrived, they would have been greeted by de León, craning their necks to take in his balding head and rough habit and, beyond him, the portico decorated with statues of the Castilian kings. As the boys were familiar with signing, they would have learned to communicate with the monk very quickly.[33] However, he focused on teaching them to speak and write rather than developing their sign language.

Two centuries later, a wealthy philanthropist, Abbé Charles-Michel de l'Épée, wandered through a poor area of Paris. He entered the house of a family he knew, and saw two little girls doing needlework, their gaze intent upon their cloth. They didn't look up when he entered.

'Good morning,' he greeted them, but they didn't respond.

He heard the rustle of skirts, and turned his head as their mother entered the room. 'Madame, your daughters are very fixed upon their work.'

'Ah, monsieur! They are deaf and dumb. They had some instruction from an elderly priest, who taught them using pictures, but he has passed on.'

Sensing a shift in the room, the two girls looked up, their eyes wide with enquiry. L'Épée, resolving that the girls must not remain ignorant of religion, learned the home signs they had developed. He enlarged and methodised their language, and made huge progress in the girls' education.[34] From 1755 to 1760 he founded L'Institut National de Jeunes Sourds de Paris, the first public school open to all deaf children.

In 1778, Samuel Heinicke opened the first institution for deaf children in Leipzig, Germany. Heinicke has since been denoted the 'father of the German method', which focused upon teaching children to speak rather than sign. These two different methods of educating children were to have massive political and social implications for deaf people as the decades passed.

Meanwhile in Britain, Thomas Braidwood established the first school for the deaf in Edinburgh in 1760 to teach deaf children to both speak and sign. American Thomas Hopkins Gallaudet visited Braidwood in 1815 to gather information on methods of deaf education. He also travelled to France to learn sign language from Abbé Roch-Ambroise Sicard, who became head of L'Institution National de Jeunes Sourds de Paris when l'Épée died. At the school in Paris, Gallaudet met Laurent Clerc, a teacher. Clerc travelled with Sicard back to America, where they then established the Hartford Asylum for the Education and Instruction of the Deaf and Dumb in America in 1817. In 1864, the National Deaf-Mute College was founded in Washington, DC. It later became known as Gallaudet University and was the first university in the world for deaf students.

Towards the end of the nineteenth century, these efforts to educate deaf people through sign language were attacked. The spread of Darwin's ideas on evolution meant that people were anxious about the distinctions between humans and animals, and speech was seen as a way of marking the divide between them.[35] Sign language was also increasingly frowned upon because it was thought to be more concrete than spoken language and unable to represent abstract concepts. As it was such a bodily language, it was thought to be more suitable for 'primitive' people or animals.

People also feared that deafness could be passed on through reproduction. Alexander Graham Bell, head of the Eugenics Section of the American Breeders Association and inventor of the telephone, was married to a woman, Mabel, who was deaf. His mother was also deaf. In 1883 he published *Memoir Upon the Formation of a Deaf Variety of the Human Race*, opening with his observations on the selective breeding of domestic animals. He suggests that 'if we could apply selection to the human race we could also produce modifications or varieties of men'.[36] This was necessary, he continues, because 'the intermarriage of congenital deaf-mutes through a number of successive generations should result in a formation of a deaf variety of the human race'.[37] As it was believed that deafness – and indeed all disabilities – could be bred out, sign language was discouraged because it enabled communication between deaf people who might otherwise fall in love and have deaf children. By contrast, oralism encouraged deaf people to mix with and marry hearing people, thereby minimising the risk of congenital deafness. However, as H-Dirksen L. Bauman, a scholar at Gallaudet University points out, less than four per cent of deaf children are born to one or more deaf parents.[38]

Speech doesn't come easily to most deaf people. For someone who is born deaf, learning to speak is a time-consuming process. Donna McDonald, author of *The Art of Being Deaf*, has been severely deaf since birth, and was taught to lip-read and speak. Her mother, she writes, 'pressed my hand against her lips so I could feel the expulsion of air shaping letters, and as she played my fingers against the pulsing of words bubbling up her throat…I was coaxed, dragooned and persuaded into the world of hearing'.[39]

Donna's words, *coaxed, dragooned, persuaded*, show how learning to speak was hardly effortless.

It's difficult to tell how much hearing Maud Praed had. Patricia Clarke quotes sections of Maud's letters in her biography of Rosa, so she was clearly literate, which suggests to me that Maud had enough hearing to pick up speech. Yet even I, who was speaking by the time I lost most of my hearing, needed frequent speech therapy when I was young. Listening, lip-reading and the anxiety of responding correctly leave me permanently exhausted. I have no doubt that it was hard for Maud, too.

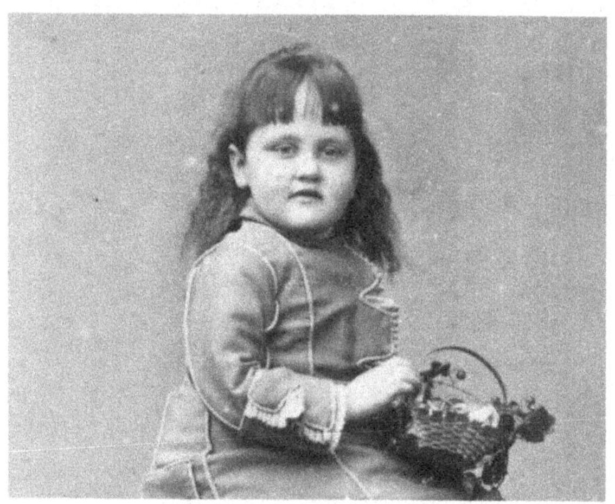

Maud at age four. John Oxley Library, State Library of Queensland, Neg No: 197579

Patricia Clarke writes that 'Rosa was fortunate to arrive in London at a time when teaching deaf people to speak, referred to as the "oral method" was spreading from the Continent'.[40] I can see how Clarke arrived at the conclusion that this was 'fortunate' timing, if one relies upon Rosa's accounts in her archives of the oral method and the evangelising of oralists (people who advocate teaching deaf people to speak rather than sign) whom she knew. But many of these accounts rarely included the voices of deaf people, and the word 'fortunate' doesn't tally with the history of deaf education.

I sense that there is something more to Maud's story, that she has been ghosted, or rendered invisible, the way I am when I can't hear enough of a conversation to join in and I stand on the edge of a group, straining for sound.

I pack my bags for Australia, but this will be a visit for launching my novel and for research, not a return.

2

Writing a Way Out

'Can you imagine what it's like to carry an idea in your head for *seven years*?' Alan Wearne, my former poetry teacher from the University of Wollongong, stands at a podium in Gleebooks bookshop in Sydney, launching my first novel, *A Curious Intimacy*. It's January 2007. Before us are my parents, my school and university friends, and my parents' friends who watched me grow up. My sister Bella has flown down from Brisbane and Oliver has come back from London. We might as well be at a wedding.

'There's a lot of drinking *tea* in this novel.' Alan has a raconteur's voice, stretching his vowels and emphasising particular words. He's already told the audience of my stubborn refusal, when I was under his tutelage, of his suggestion to remove the word *gleam* from a poem. The room glows with laughter, bright faces and clapping as he launches my first novel. My breath, shallow with anxiety and excitement, slows. I am exactly where I am supposed to be, and it was deafness that drew me here.

~

If my first memory is of the ache of meningitis and the shiver of the apricot tree's leaves, my second is of Dad reading to me from the Strawberry Shortcake book on my hospital bed. I couldn't hear him, but the book took the place of his voice, the illustrations absorbing me.

When I was better, and back at home, Dad read to Bella, Oliver and me before we switched out the light for sleep. He lay on Oliver's trundle bed and we piled on top of him. I sprawled halfway across his chest and felt the vibrations of his voice travelling through our skin. The book we'd picked was an underwater adventure story, with blanks in the sentences for character names so that he could use ours.

'Jessica floated into the deep blue sea in her submarine.'

'Does it really have my name in there?' I clambered up to peer at the pages.

'No.'

I sank back down, disappointed.

On my first day at school, Mum and Dad were travelling in India; they needed a holiday by then. Mum's parents, Jean and John, moved from New Zealand to the farm for three months to take care of Bella, Oliver and me. Jean drove me to school on my first day. On the cement pavement by the school's entrance, I stood beside her as she spoke to my teacher. I craned my head back to watch them, willing myself not to cry.

Two decades later, over lunch in the Botanical Gardens at Christchurch, Jean told me that whenever I stepped off the bus, 'Your shoelaces were undone, your plaits were unravelling and your schoolbag was sliding off your shoulder, but in your hand you had a book.'

She was less impressed when we reached home and I threw my bag against the wall of the verandah.

'Hang it up on the hook.'

I bolted outside to play with Oliver.

'When I asked you to do something you didn't want to do,' Jean told me in the gardens, 'you gave me the dirtiest look.'

In Kindergarten I sat next to Ruby, who had pale skin, freckles and thick black hair. Sometimes I pulled out a tall book Mum had given me. It was padded with pop-out dinosaurs and illustrated with cavemen in their homes, which were protected by rough wooden fortresses. I stood the book upright on my desk and hid my head in it until the teacher came along.

'Put that away and do your letters,' she said. 'Watch what Ruby's doing.'

I glanced at Ruby's exercise book, envious of her round, tidy *a*s and *b*s. Reluctantly, I closed my dinosaur book, feeling exposed.

When I learned to read, I learned to escape. Instead of trying to join in on conversations and becoming frustrated because I could never hear enough, I submerged myself in other worlds. I swam with Erika to underwater islands in *My Sister Sif*, danced with Emma Macalik Butterworth in *As the Waltz Was Ending*, and followed Mrs Danvers down the hall in Daphne du Maurier's *Rebecca*, the air thick with Rebecca's absence. When I was reading, my deafness was irrelevant. The characters asked nothing of me, only swept me up into their dramas and excursions.

Sometimes I read so obsessively that Mum became exasperated. 'Put your book down and go out and talk to people!' she exhorted as I nestled in a beanbag, a book open in my lap. Her visitors sat around the table next to me, drinking tea and eating Anzac biscuits. Outside, their children ran on the grass.

I frowned. She seemed not to understand how difficult it was for me to join in on their games. In later years, I realised she was concerned that, if I never overcame my shyness, I wouldn't be able to get ahead.

Reading filled in long trips on the bus to school, in the car to piano or flute lessons, or to the audiologist, or to holidays in Sydney or on the coast. The skin of my left cheek, always exposed to the sun in the passenger seat, was stippled with more freckles than my right.

It isn't so surprising, then, that from reading, which was bound up with travelling and which took me to other places, I made a leap to writing.

Every week when I was young, Mum wrote a letter to her mother in Christchurch, her square cursive marching across the thin airmail paper she used to save on postage. From age seven I copied her, sending letters to my grandmother, her sister and my mother's sister, all in Christchurch. During school holidays I wrote to friends from school, my support teacher Mrs Matthews, and friends of my parents. Yet this network of readers wasn't enough.

When I was ten, Mum and Dad squashed Bella, Oliver and me into the back of our red Commodore and drove for eight hours until we reached Expo 88 in Brisbane. Wearing Ken Done T-shirts, we queued outside tall gates beside the river. Once we finally filed inside, we were overwhelmed. We travelled on a monorail for the first time, our faces squished against the window as we looked out at the wide span of the Brisbane River. Creatures on stilts in shimmering pants and butterfly wings stepped among the crowds. A cart on a track took us through a strip of Queensland rainforest, and Mum bought a spicy serving of Nepalese food from the pagodas. It gave her diarrhoea, just as it had when she'd travelled to Nepal five years before.

Outside the Australia Post pavilion stood several tall tubes fitted with computer screens. I watched as people pressed a button on the tube, which then spat out a postcard. On the card was the name and address of a person who wanted a penpal. Desperate to expand my collection of correspondents, I pressed the button three times and received two penpals from Singapore and one from America.

Back on the farm, I pulled out my stationery collection patterned with flowers and leaves, and wrote three letters. With the American and one of the girls in Singapore I exchanged only one letter, but the other Singaporean and I carried on a correspondence for years. I loved printing her lengthy, elaborate address on an envelope and receiving her replies on small, precisely folded pieces of notepaper.

Are there any farms in Singapore?

No, there's not enough space for farms, only parks.

I could not fathom this: how did Singaporeans eat?

I sensed that money was tight for my friend, for she lived in a small apartment with her parents and sister. Although my parents were frugal and my brother, sister and I knew not to ask for frivolous things, I had my first inkling of how privileged we were because we were surrounded by space. Letters opened my life, isolated as it was by deafness and the distance of country living.

As we were so far out of town, we posted mail by leaving it on the shelf of our mailbox, an old white petrol drum on a stand on the main road. The mailman came on Mondays, Wednesdays and Fridays to collect and drop off our letters. During the holidays I walked or cycled down our dusty gravel road to check if the postie had left anything. If there was a letter addressed to me, I'd tuck the bills for Mum and Dad under my arm and examine the stamps and postmark to see if it was from Australia, New Zealand or Singapore. If I was able to wait until I reached home, I sat on the verandah at the old school desk that Dad had salvaged, lifted its sloping lid and fished out my letter opener with the piece of green and grey speckled paua shell pressed into its handle. Mum had bought it for me in New Zealand.

More often, I opened the letter as I walked, sun burning the nape of my neck, reading my grandmother's account of the drought in New Zealand that made the butter taste strange because the dairy cows were feeding on grain, or of my Singaporean friend's school lessons. By the time I reached our house and climbed over the fence into the front garden, I was glowing with pleasure.

The letters I wrote to my relatives and penpals were my earliest forays into writing. They were an unthreatening way for me to make connections and to satisfy my desire – still then unknown to me – for people's company. Perhaps this was the reason why, in my late teens and early twenties at university, I identified so strongly with the letters of nineteenth-century women writers such as Rachel Henning and Georgiana Molloy. They, too, waited impatiently, often for months at a time, for conversations to continue between sheaves of paper. They depended upon letters to provide social nourishment and to eclipse the vast distance between England and Australia, which was not unlike the distance between me and other people.

The National Library of Canberra holds some of Maud's letters in her family's archive, the Murray-Prior Papers. I'm keen to read what Maud wrote so I can see what her life was like and how deafness impacted upon it. After my launch in Sydney, I book a flight to the nation's capital.

~

The colours of Canberra are similar to those of London, but the city is quieter, almost ghostly, the place's energy dispersed across the surface of Lake Burley Griffin. I head from the lake up to the library's steps, pausing to gaze across the Patrick White Lawns.

I wonder what it was like for White, coming back after the Second World War to a conservative country with his partner Manoly, raising goats on the outskirts of Sydney to make a living. It must have been difficult, if he referred in his essay 'The Prodigal Son' to 'the Great Australian Emptiness, in which the mind is the least of possessions'.[1] Yet he endured cultural isolation so that he could be in Australia again. I think of my own persistent homesickness, and sympathise.

Inside the library I head to the Special Collections reading room and pick up the first box I've ordered. The Murray-Prior Papers include letters, documents, journals and photographs that belonged to Rosa and her father Thomas Murray-Prior, her stepmother Nora, people related to the Murray-Prior family by marriage, and Rosa's companion Nancy Harward. The material constitutes roughly half of Rosa's archive; the other half is in the State Library of Queensland.

I work solidly through letters, diaries and photographs, using a finding aid created by Colin Roderick, who wrote the first biography on Rosa.[2] When I come to Maud's letters, I study them closely.

The handwriting of her early letters is neat and clear. Having watched her mother write novels, Maud understood the process of redrafting and, given that her writing is so careful in some letters, it's likely she wrote drafts, then fair copies, of her letters. I photograph them on my digital camera so that I can transcribe them later.

As I read, I gather an impression of Maud as an inquisitive, observant child. To her grandmother Nora she described a holiday she took by the seaside with her father and brothers when she was thirteen. There was a forest 'with a church in the middle of it' that had once existed on the shore but had been cut down and 'when the tide is very low, we might see some stumps of the trees'.[3] Maud also noticed the seasons. To Nora she wrote, 'the leaves will soon fall and winter will come with Christmas'.[4] To her aunts Meta and Dorothy she complained that her brother Geoffrey 'has been collecting some birds' eggs and butterflies. It seems cruel of him to kill such little creatures.'[5] In a letter of 1886 she recounted an excursion to the Natural History Museum where she saw 'a great many capital foreign things', including 'two large monkeys head [sic] in bottles, they looked nasty and smashed'.[6]

I imagine Maud walking to the museum, then a fairly new building that had opened its doors five years before. Her companion would have held her hand as they crossed the road so Maud wouldn't be hit by a horse and carriage she couldn't hear. Perhaps, at the entrance to the stately terracotta building, Maud's companion would face her so that Maud could read her lips as she explained what they would be seeing and how long it would take. Inside, Maud might have felt the cool air of the large Hintze Hall on her cheeks, or looked up to admire the panels painted with images of plants from across the globe.

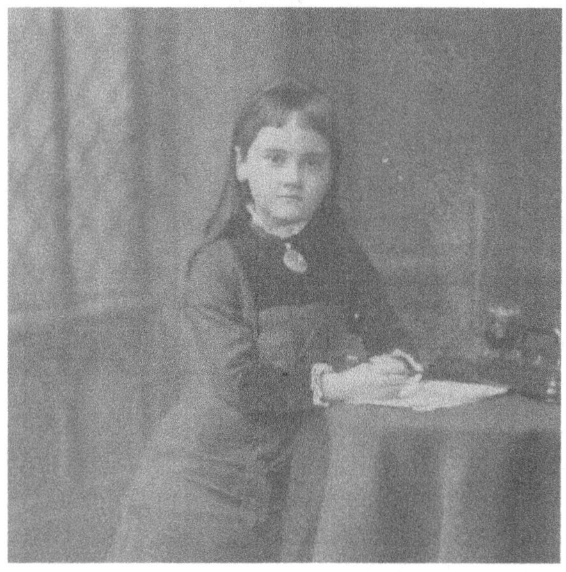

Maud as a young girl with pen in hand. John Oxley Library, State Library of Queensland, Neg No: 18492

Maud used her writing to connect with people. Her later letters in particular, written when she was around fifteen and older, dispense with her dutiful tone and show a natural desire to socialise. Of her aunts Meta and Dorothy, she asked, 'Please do write to me and tell me about yourselves.'[7] She wrote assiduously to her brother Humphrey, her second younger brother, who travelled from England to Western Australia to become a mine manager before moving to the orchards of San Francisco. In an undated missive, Humphrey wrote, 'Thanks awfully for your letter which gave me more news than any. Please write often.'[8]

Always at home, Maud was able to pass on information about the family easily. Humphrey wrote, 'I receive the papers regularly and also your letters',[9] which suggests that she corresponded frequently. Maud loved her family and wanted to be in touch with them.

The clarity of Maud's writing also suggests that she had enough hearing to learn to speak, read and write. Perhaps this is why Rosa decided to enrol her daughter in Benjamin St John Ackers' school, which focused upon oralism, or teaching deaf children to speak rather than sign. The school was never large. In 1887 there were seventeen children, in 1895 there were fourteen, and in 1907 there were six.[10]

When Ackers came to the school, it was run by Susannah Hull, who was passionate about oralism. Hull, the daughter of a doctor, became interested in teaching one of her father's patients who had become deaf and blind from scarlet fever. In 1862 she opened a school in a room in her father's house, intending to teach children who had acquired speech before they lost their hearing. When she discovered in her reading that children who had been deaf since birth could be taught to speak, she began to teach these children as well.[11]

In 1868, Hull asked for help from Alexander Melville Bell in America to adapt his method of Visible Speech to her school.[12] In this system, a written shape corresponded to a sound that was found in speech. The system was used to teach people how to speak a language they had not heard before, such as Sanskrit. It was also used to teach deaf people to speak by shaping their mouths according the symbols. Alexander Melville Bell was too busy to come, so he sent his son Alexander Graham Bell, then twenty-one years old. Alexander, whose mother Eliza was deaf, was raised in a family that was dedicated to speech: his grandfather lectured on speech disorders and phonetics; his father lectured on elocution and philology; and his uncle was a professor of elocution and English literature.

Bell's excursion to London to help Susannah Hull learn his father's technique of visible speech was revolutionary. He wrote, 'I went to Miss Hull's school to assist her in making the experiment, and was thus introduced to what proved to be my life-work – the teaching of speech to the deaf.'[13] Teaching deaf students prompted him to study the vibrations in air as speech was uttered, 'with the object of developing an apparatus that would enable my deaf pupils to see and recognise the forms of vibration characteristic of the various elements of speech'. His experiments in this area 'paved the way for the appearance of the first membrane telephone, the ancestor of all the telephones of today'.[14] In 1872, Bell set up his own school in Boston. One of his pupils was Helen Keller, the famous blind and deaf scholar. All this time, Bell was working on inventions that would transmit the human voice, and the telephone was patented in the United States in 1876.

Bell described Hull, who was zealous in her beliefs that deaf children should be taught to speak, as 'the great pioneer of oral teaching in England'.[15] In an 1877 essay, 'Do Persons Born Deaf Differ Mentally from Others Who Have the Power of Hearing?' Hull wrote:

> Spoken language is the product of ages – the workmanship of many minds; one of the cornerstones of civilization and the crown of history. Indeed, without it, history, such as we have it, could never

> have been. When, therefore, we give our deaf children a sign-language, we give them an instrument for expressing their thoughts, but a very poor and feeble one. We push them back in the world's history to the infancy of our race. They may, as French-system teachers love to boast, be understood, to some extent, by American Indians and other savage tribes![16]

The words Hull uses to describe sign language reveal the common belief that it was too simple to encompass concepts – it is a *poor* and *feeble instrument*. It's a language used by races that people once considered to be primitive – *American Indians* and *savage tribes*. It is further down in the evolutionary chain because it belongs to the *infancy of our race*. The influence of social Darwinism, which was in vogue at this time, is clear.

Hull's words give me a clue to another reason why Rosa chose to teach her daughter to speak: she, too, was obsessed with ideas of racial hierarchy. In her 1902 novel *Fugitive Anne*, Rosa's protagonist Anne escapes from her violent husband of four months by jumping from the steamer that is carrying them to London. With her is her faithful manservant Kombo, her Aboriginal childhood friend. Kombo is described as 'well tamed, having been taken young from his tribe', a reference to the forcible removal of Aboriginal children from their families from the late nineteenth century to the 1970s, and their assimilation into white culture. When Kombo set out to find his family, he 'would cast off the garments of civilisation and relapse into his original condition of barbarism'.[17] His culture and language are referred to in terms that suggest primitivism, an impression reinforced by the contrast between the 'magic' of Anne's voice when she sings in her 'glorious contralto in a hymn' and Kombo's broken English. The imagery is clear: to speak well is to belong, in Rosa's terms, to a higher race.

Like Aboriginal people, deaf people in the late nineteenth century were encouraged to assimilate into the dominant culture (in this case, hearing culture) through marriage, due to anxiety about congenital deafness. Rosa discussed her fears that Maud's deafness could be inherited with her friend Eliza Lynn Linton, a journalist and fellow author. Linton wrote to Rosa about 'two deaf and dumb people who married…and they were perfectly happy', although she didn't know whether their children were deaf, which, she added, 'would depend on whether the deafness were by heredity or had been caused by a damaging at the birth.'[18] Linton's reference to a happy deaf couple suggests she thought it would be good for Maud to make other deaf friends, and perhaps even find a deaf husband. She must have recognised how lonely Maud was, for she suggested when Maud was in her early twenties, 'I wonder how it would be if you had a deaf & dumb companion for her? – whether they would feel more companionship together than she with one who had all her senses? It might be that she would feel a greater harmony of condition – more solidarity of life & functions.'[19] Rosa, however, remained committed to teaching Maud to speak and to raising her among hearing people.

Although Rosa and Campbell were already generous donors to Maud's school, in 1884 Rosa edited a volume of essays and poetry, *For Their Sakes*, to raise more funds. Rosa's introduction to the volume confirms how important it was to her that Maud learned to speak:

> What joy when the child can read from the lips of those around – when it can ask questions and

> understand the answers! What a different place the world, a little while ago so dreary, seems now to the poor little wondering thing! The mournful face begins to brighten; games and laughter are no longer meaningless; the closed mind gradually unfolds; the struggling thoughts find vent; and the active brain reasons. It is as though a great wall had been knocked down: silence and solitude upon one side; companionship, sympathy, interest – all that makes life worth living – on the other.[20]

Rosa sets up a contrast between light and dark, mournfulness and brightness, dumbness and intelligence. She suggests that a deaf child who cannot speak has no access to language, and that they are, as many people such as Hull once thought them, imbecilic.

These negative connotations of deafness reappear in an essay by Benjamin St John Ackers, which Rosa included in her volume. He wrote that, 'If the deaf are unable to mix comfortably with hearing persons, they will naturally shrink from them; be drawn to others like themselves; marry those similarly afflicted and so, alas, too often hand down and increase the evil.'[21] If deafness corresponded with animality for writers such as Alexander Graham Bell, for Benjamin St John Ackers it meant criminality and corruption.

In 1880 the oral method of teaching deaf children was cemented by a gathering of educators for the deaf known as the Milan Conference. It was arranged by the Pereira Society, an organisation founded by the grandson of Jacob Rodrigues Pereira (1715–80), a teacher for the deaf. Just as Benjamin St John Ackers established the Society for Training Teachers of the Deaf and the Diffusion of the 'German' System, so too was the Pereira Society established to promote and disperse the oral method of teaching deaf children to speak.[22]

At the Milan conference, twelve speakers presented on education for deaf children. Of these, nine spoke in support of oralism, including the head of Maud's school, Benjamin St John Ackers; his wife; the principal, Arthur Kinsey; vice-principal Susannah Hull; and David Buxton, the secretary of the Society for Training Teachers of the Deaf and the Diffusion of the 'German' System. No deaf people were involved in putting forth or voting for the resolution to ban the teaching of sign language in favour of oralism, but from these biased proceedings the motion was passed.

The ramifications of this conference were profound: for the next century deaf people were forced to communicate in a difficult language, for which they were often mocked because they could not hear themselves well enough to speak. Teachers who taught sign language lost their jobs, and the solidarity and culture that deaf communities provided was eroded, particularly as these communities were formed in schools.

The impact was also felt by Ackers' daughter. Her father had maintained, in a paper titled 'Advantages to the Deaf of the "German" System in After Life', that 'even the *toto-congenital* deaf taught by articulation do not forget when they leave school the chief part of the learning acquired there' – that is, when they finished their education.[23]

Ackers died in 1915. In 1932, Reverend F.W.G. Gilby, whose deaf parents signed, paid Ackers' daughter a visit. In his autobiography he wrote,

> I found [Ackers'] poor deaf daughter living in loneliness in Taunton not too good a lip reader or

> even specially good as an articulator of speech. She was living almost alone, and afraid of me as a stranger when I paid my first visit to her pretty little home. She used a slate to converse with me, and I was not asked to sit down, and had to leave very soon. On the next occasion shortly after she had more courage and I was allowed to sit down, and we talked, on a third visit we were even less constrained and I invited her to my services for the deaf and dumb in Taunton, she unfroze rapidly after that and attended quite often and once remarked 'What would my Father have said!'...People who could hear had not troubled to give her any conversation that was worth calling by that name.[24]

A lifetime of championing oralism, and it had come to this: a terrible, unabated loneliness.

~

Maud became a boarder at her school because her parents moved to Northamptonshire, some hundred kilometres from London. Rosa's father, Thomas Murray-Prior, visited England in 1882. With Rosa, he called on Maud at Ealing. In the schoolroom, he kissed his granddaughter in greeting, noting that she had black eyes, thick brown hair, and her mother's and grandmother's chin. He looked at the classroom of wide-eyed children, their bodies poised with attention. On the board were a list of sounds that were difficult to pronounce, such as *Sha-Scha*.

The teacher called on a boy from South America, tapping on his desk. To Murray-Prior, he looked intelligent, with dark, lively eyes. Murray-Prior listened as the boy spoke the sounds written on the board.

'What is this?' The teacher touched the chair.

'This is a chair,' the boy replied.

'Che-Kà,' the teacher wrote on the board. She made the boy repeat the word until his pronunciation was correct.

Maud was summoned to stand. She twisted from side to side with excitement, reciting her three-times table and answering questions from a picture her teacher held up. When she wrote the answers on the board, her handwriting was plain and clear.

Murray-Prior bent before one of the boys and asked, 'How old are you?'

The boy frowned in puzzlement and the teacher appeared at his side. 'Your moustache is too thick,' he told Murray-Prior.

Murray-Prior lifted up the hair from his mouth so the boy could see his lips. 'Do you read any historical books?'

The boy tried to form the word 'historical', and with the teacher's help he made it out. His forehead smoothed with relief.

At the end of the visit, Murray-Prior left with his daughter. As they walked out, he said, 'It's sad, my dear Rosie, for Maudie is so bright. She would have been very accomplished.'

'Yes.'

'But she is a darling little creature, and speaking so well.'[25]

Maud was eight years old at the time of this visit, and she must have missed her mother terribly. Thomas Murray-Prior observed that she was 'quite delighted to see her Mother' and he 'did not like keeping her from Mamma'.

Rosa's stepsister Lizzie, who came to visit not long after the Praeds moved to England, wrote to her father that Maud 'began to explain in her pretty way how she had been to school but now she was home and did not want to leave again'.[26] In another letter, written a month later, Lizzie added that Maud seemed 'happy and content at school which is a great comfort'.[27] Perhaps it was the contact with her mother that reminded Maud of what she was missing.

In school holidays, Rosa employed Maud's teacher Elizabeth Frances Boultbee as a companion. Elizabeth had learned lip-reading to teach her younger sister Anne, who was deaf. When Anne died at age twenty-two in 1867, Elizabeth began teaching a broader group of children, including Maud. In 1902, the same year Rosa published *Fugitive Anne*, Elizabeth published *Practical Lip-Reading for the Use of the Deaf.* Like other oralists, she decried sign language and lauded lip-reading. She wrote that 'the Lip-Reader cannot but rejoice when intelligent thought overcomes prejudice, and each fresh blow is gradually shattering that old worn-out system which only binds the poor deaf mute the more closely with the cruel shackles of solitude and misery'.[28] Again, sign language is laden with such negative associations as *worn-out* and *cruel.*

Many of the teachers who instructed children in lip-reading were women, and Maud would have become accustomed to a female presence near her, whether it was her mother or a teacher. The smell and smoothness of their skin, their routines in dressing, and the particularities of their expressions were a constant in her days.

~

Most, if not all, children fear separation from their parents, but my terror was magnified by my deafness. If my parents called out, I might not be able to hear them, and even if I could hear them, I wouldn't be able to tell where the sound was coming from.

At the Royal Easter Show in Sydney when I was eight, I stopped in the crowd to look up at a plane writing in the sky. Among the bodies pressing into me, I lost track of Mum, who was wearing a pink plastic top hat from my Pink Panther showbag. I knew roughly which way she'd gone, and soon found her staring about with wild-eyed panic.

'What if I couldn't find you, Mum?' I asked as she grabbed my sweaty hand. 'What would I do?'

'We'd ask them to make an announcement over the loudspeakers.'

'But I wouldn't be able to hear the loudspeakers.'

'Then you'd find an adult, explain to them that you're deaf, and they'll find us.'

I kept close to my family for the rest of that day.

When I was seven, I stood before the microphone at school assembly, my exercise book gripped in my hands. Before me, a hundred kids sat cross-legged on the floor. Two hundred eyes watched me expectantly.

'Lost in the bush,' I announced. Swaying slightly, I read out a story about bushwalking with my parents. We had stopped to look up at a bird in the trees above, but when I glanced down Mum and Dad had gone. Panic engulfed me. I followed the track around a bench in the bush and, to my relief, I saw them ahead.

'The end,' I finished. As the school clapped dutifully, I sat down, aglow. It was my first brush with literary fame.

More importantly, it was a way of expressing my fears, which I was too young to analyse. Two years after I wrote my bush story, I described my parents going to New Zealand, leaving me behind on the farm. I copied the story into my exercise book in my large, awkward handwriting and gave it to Mrs Matthews.

After she read the story, Mrs Matthews spoke to my mother and my mother talked to me. Mum reiterated, 'We will never, ever leave you.'

~

In the reading room at the National Library, my back aches from standing and taking photographs all day. Before me, on a slanted book rest, is Maud's journal. It's a stiff-backed book covered in red marbled paper. Maud wrote in the journal to record her impression of her 1894 trip with her mother to Australia, Singapore, Hong Kong, Japan and Canada. Maud might have written a journal for each country, but the only extant one relates to Japan.

Maud's handwriting is faded, but still legible. She describes an American widow who 'proudly held a dark brown silk embroidered parasol over her head. She wore a grey crepe dress for climbing! We were carried in sedan chairs with four coolies each. As they laboured up the mountains, they mopped their faces with their handkerchiefs.'[29] I assume that Maud recounted these incidents so that her mother could later draw on them for 'copy' or material for her books, as was her habit. But Rosa might also have used the journal to prompt Maud to engage with the world around her and to build her confidence, as she did with Maud's art.

In the summer of 1890, when the family stayed at Rushden, near Wellingborough where Campbell worked in the brewery,

Maud took lessons from Mortimer Menpes, an Australian artist born in Adelaide. He moved to London when he was twenty and was taught by James McNeill Whistler, who became a godfather for his second child. In a letter to her grandfather Thomas Murray-Prior, Maud described how Menpes 'wrote down about the colours for me, and put them on my palette in successive order… and placed some black and white rags on the lawn on which we gazed from the terrace. They helped me to see the difference between the dark and light colours.'[30]

Menpes had a huge handlebar moustache that covered his lips, and it would have been difficult for Maud to lip-read him. Perhaps he spoke to Rosa, who repeated what he said to Maud. The girl would have transferred her gaze from their lips to the palette of colours, to the lawn, to the easel.

Occasionally Maud used her mother as a subject. To her aunt Dorothy, she wrote, 'I have been doing a highly finished pencil drawing of Mother typewriting in her boudoir…Everybody who sees it says that it is an excellent likeness of her. Father wants to have it printed in "Black and White." It would be rather an honour for me.'[31] *Black and White* was an illustrated weekly periodical founded in 1891 by Charles Norris Williamson. It featured stories by Arthur Conan Doyle, Henry James, Bram Stoker, H.G. Wells and Jerome K. Jerome. A number of Maud's drawings were published in this magazine, although it's not clear if this particular drawing was printed.[32]

Among the sheaves of paper in the National Library of Australia, I find Maud's pen-and-ink drawing of her mother. Rosa's face is calm, almost regal, her hair coiled on her head, her neck and left cheek set off by a richly embroidered jacket. The outlines of her face are simple, in contrast to the thick detail of her hair and clothes. Perhaps this was a reflection of Maud's relationship to her mother, for that face was the most familiar thing she knew, and the most steady source of information about her days. An accompanying note explains the drawing was made when Maud was twenty-four, in 1896.[33]

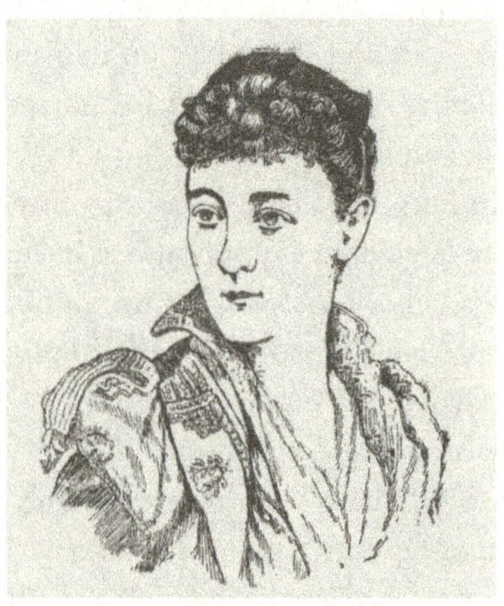

Maud's drawing of her mother, Rosa. Murray-Prior Papers, Box 3, Folder 22, 19/63, National Library of Australia

Art boosted Maud's sense of assurance and gave her something to focus on. It could be taught to her relatively easily, given that lessons were delivered individually or in small groups. As well as writing during the trip in Japan, Maud kept up with her sketching. She wrote in her journal:

> June 11th A sweet looking Japanese nesan looked after our luggage and attended to Mother's wants. I took my sketch book out of the 'Cannes' bag; I made a sign saying sketch her. She cheerfully nodded. Her eyes

> were loving & expressive. Her lips were curved & sad. She was a dear little woman much shorter than I was. Oh that we could have her for a servant in England. I bid her perch on Mother's bed, oh I loved her – she moved her face upright, her hair was like that of an inexperienced demoiselle. She looked happy – she watched mother's stylographic pen as Mother was writing by the Bow window. When the sketch was done, she seized it and nodded sympathetically.[34]

This piece of writing shows how, at twenty-two, Maud was confident enough to engage with someone quite different from herself. It demonstrates her attentiveness to body language: the woman's countenance, her lips, and where she directed her gaze. As someone who couldn't hear, Maud would have relied on reading body language to work out what people were saying or thinking. It shows her belonging to a family of artists – she draws while her mother writes – and perhaps her aspiration to become one as well. Her mention of appropriating the woman as a servant also shows she has adopted some of her mother's racist attitudes. Never independent from her family and teachers, Maud readily absorbed their ideas.

Above all, Maud's art was an escape. To her grandfather, she described it thus: 'The work keeps me away from all the trifling troubles and is the only consolation in my life.'[35] Maud's intense concentration on the purely visual aspects of line, colour and movement would have been a respite from the constant strain of listening and of trying to work out what was happening around her.

~

In the early 1980s Mum, who was fascinated by technology, bought a Commodore 64 computer. While my brother and male cousins clustered around it like flies to play *Parallax* and *Caveman Ugh-lympics*, the cane chair creaking as they swerved from side to side with their avatars, I taught myself touch-typing and typed up my stories.

Mum owned a typewriter on which she'd typed letters to my father, but she forbade me from using it. 'You'll jam the keys.'

When the computer arrived, I pestered her, 'Can we have a printer, too, please Mum? You never let me use the typewriter.'

She finally agreed and I hovered as she unpacked the box on the dining-room table and pulled out the dot-matrix printer. When it was plugged in, I began writing stories in earnest. I rewrote fairy tales, inverting them, so that Little Red Riding Hood was a horrible child and her grandmother was pleased when the wolf ate her up. I liked this approach because of the intellectual joy of taking apart and replacing plot points, and of seeing what pulling at the structure would do.

I also wrote these kinds of stories because, on some level, I recognised that I couldn't be part of a conventional narrative. In most of the books I read, children rescued dogs, fought dragons and wrote letters to their sweethearts. I couldn't do any of these things without help, and my chances of finding a sweetheart were slim given my unease with communicating. Instead I wrote how the prince found Sleeping Beauty a bore because she hadn't done anything except sleep for a century.

At school I showed my stories to Mrs Matthews. After she read them, she came up with the idea of putting together a magazine. 'This will teach you some interviewing skills. We'll go to the police station so you can interview the sergeant.'

'Okay.'

My brother was friends with the sergeant's son, and Dad had visited the station to get his gun licence for shooting roos, so I wasn't too anxious. Even so, looking at the large man on the other side of the wide desk in the police station, I was glad to have Mrs Matthews next to me. In his stiff, dark-blue uniform, fingers knitted across his stomach, the sergeant answered the questions I'd workshopped with Mrs Matthews. After the interview, he showed us around the station, stopping by a tray of seedlings.

I stared. 'What are they for?'

He exchanged a smile with Mrs Matthews and moved us on. It would be years before I worked out that they were tiny marijuana plants.

I typed up my article on our computer, found some stories in my writing folder and drew some pictures. I glued these onto sheets of paper, which Mrs Matthews photocopied in the staff room, handing them to me to staple at the table. We distributed the magazine to the staff, my parents and relatives. Watching them turn the pages, I exploded with pride.

~

The State Library of Queensland contains the other half of Rosa's archives. This building isn't conventional, or box-like. It takes advantage of the city's subtropical climate and exposes parts of itself to the elements. The central court is covered by a roof over the fifth floor, while the outdoor lounge of the adjacent café is protected from rain by the floor above. The wireless signal is strong enough to reach users wandering with their mobiles, or sitting with their laptops on a cement slab outside the café, or in tiny alcoves with desks on each floor. In each of these alcoves is an image by Badtjala artist Fiona Foley that explores how opium was given to Aboriginal people in Queensland as payment for their labour. It ruined their health and, sometimes, their lives.

I'm here after my stint in Canberra and I'm glad of the warmer weather. Rosa's archives are on the fourth floor in the John Oxley Library. When I reach the reading room I'm dazzled by sunlight flooding through the glass walls. I wait for my eyes to adjust, then take in the view of Maiwar, the milky brown river shaded by trees. Tall office towers rise behind it.

I collect the box of archives I ordered the night before and pull on a pair of white cotton gloves. As with the Murray-Prior Papers in the National Library of Australia, there's a vast amount of material – some twenty-five boxes of it – including Rosa's letters, ideas for stories, newspaper clippings and transcripts of communication with the dead. In an exercise book is a rough draft of *The Romance of Mademoiselle Aïssé*, published in 1910. Handwritten pages are held together with now-rusty pins. At the top of one is the note, 'This page not to be typed.' An envelope with 'The British Empire Hotel' logo in the upper left corner lies loose among the pages, addressed to *Mrs Campbell Praed, The Westbourne Hotel, Duke Street, Bath.* Another opened envelope, dated *Feb 17, 6-PM,* is stamped with a postmark titled 'British Industries Fair Textiles at White City, London 1932'. The texture and detail of these papers make me feel closer to Rosa. In her notes, annotations, the paraphernalia of letter writing, I see the imprint of her personality: capacious, curious and able to absorb tranches of emotion.

The sheer volume of material is bewildering and, to my relief, there's a finding aid for each of the boxes. I scan it for mentions of Maud, and find she appears in letters that her brothers Bulkley and Humphrey wrote to their mother. I order some of Bulkley's letters.

In 1887, Campbell Praed's friend William Knox D'Arcy moved to England with his family. D'Arcy had been a solicitor in Rockhampton while Campbell was living on Curtis Island, and became enormously wealthy through share trading and mining interests. Two years after his arrival in England, D'Arcy installed his family at Stanmore Hall, a sprawling Tudor-style mansion north-west of London.[36] Bulkley attended Westminster School in London with the D'Arcy boys Frank and Lionel, and the Praed and D'Arcy children grew to know one another well.[37]

At Stanmore Hall, D'Arcy hosted grand balls that the Praeds attended. Bulkley wrote to his mother that 'we had ripping fun at Stanmore, and I think Maud enjoyed herself as well'.[38] At one ball, however, his sister's behaviour disconcerted him.

As I scan Bulkley's letter, I see Maud standing close to him in a large room full of people. The light from the gas lamps isn't bright enough to read lips by, especially as people talk quickly with excitement. Instead Maud watches women in extravagant gowns with cap sleeves and scooped necklines, their skirts swaying and trains trailing. She smells perfume, sweat and the oil from men's hair, and feels the patter of shoes on the floor as people dance. Light shines on women's bare chests and refracts through their diamond earrings as they tilt their heads, laughing. No one catches her eye as they pass.

A couple approach Bulkley, who stands erect with his hands clasped behind his back. His hair, parted down the centre, is smoothed flat, his thick moustache neatly trimmed. He leans forward, his face pleasant, and extends his hand to them.

Maud watches his mouth. 'This is Maud.'

She turns her head to the couple. 'I'm pleased to meet you.'

They stare at her. Maud takes in their wide eyes and furrowed brow, the way they smile and move on.

'Why does not everybody dance with me? Why do they look at me like that when they are introduced?' she asks Bulkley.

'That's tommyrot, Maud. You don't know what you're talking about. Come on, let's dance.'

When the dance finishes, Bulkley sees Lena D'Arcy, the eldest D'Arcy daughter. He guides Maud towards the dark-haired, pretty young woman. After talking to Bulkley, Lena takes Maud's arm and leads her through the crowd, making sure she looks at Maud when speaking. They pile their plates with small cakes at the back of the room and sit on velvet-covered chairs to eat them. When Maud's plate is clear of crumbs and cream, she gravitates back to Bulkley.[39]

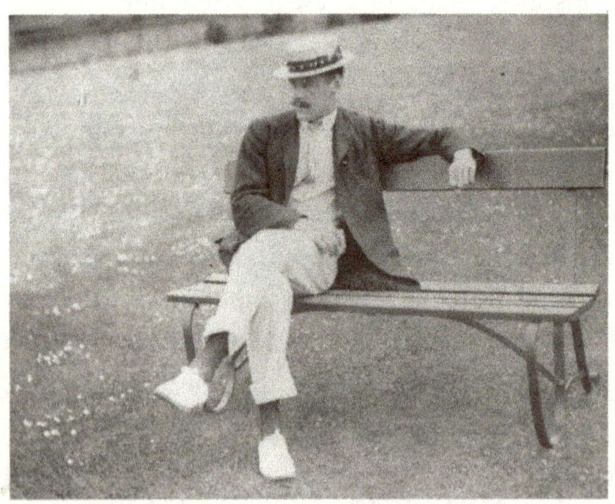

Bulkley Praed. John Oxley Library, State Library of Queensland, Neg No: 124268

Rosa's biographer Patricia Clarke writes that Maud's conduct, or whatever had caused the people at the ball to stare at her, suggested 'signs of awkwardness and eccentric behaviour in social situations', where previously Maud had been 'an apparently well-adjusted, attractive young woman coping well with the disability of deafness'.[40] To me, Maud's awkwardness reads as the fairly routine expression of a deaf person trying to communicate but not getting it right by a hearing person's standards. Maud's voice, for example, might have been pitched too loudly or too high, for she wouldn't have had enough hearing to regulate it. She might simply have misheard a question and not given the expected answer.

Clarke describes Bulkley as 'admittedly an easily embarrassed observer',[41] and at eighteen he may not have had much appreciation for the complexities of his sister's disability. He believed that the best thing for Maud was to keep her away from all social contact, suggesting to his father that 'it is an awful mistake letting her go to these things at all' even though 'she seems awfully happy on the top of it and likes being there immensely'.[42] To Bulkley it was unfathomable 'how she can like society under those circumstances... Wouldn't it simplify matters if she didn't.'[43] Their father agreed after the dance that Maud would 'have to make a break for it some time or other; why not break at once and not give her a taste for it', but, Bulkley complained to his mother, 'you know what it is, the next invitation that Maud gets, he'll accept like a shot'.[44]

It's clear from these letters that Maud enjoyed socialising. Humphrey, the second-eldest brother, commented on her busy social life in a letter: 'The hot weather is just starting again and consequently I am feeling very far from energetic; with you of course weather & feeling are just the reverse. The latter is plainly visible from the number of visits you seem to be paying.'[45] It was hard at times, however, for Maud to get the knack of social nuances.

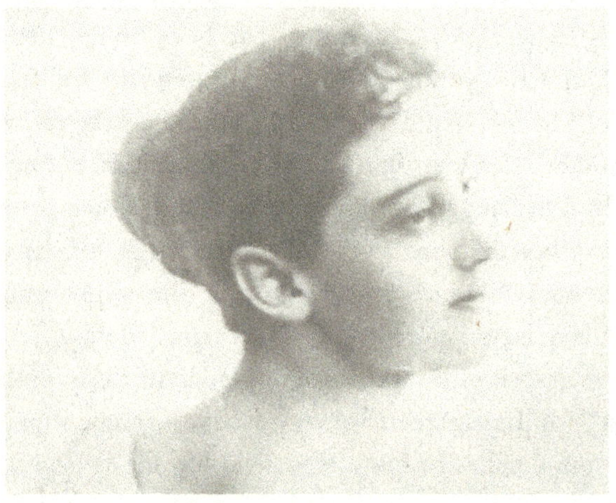

Maud age twenty-one. State Library of NSW, PXA 1403

~

At age thirteen, I agreed to go to a party at a shed on a nearby farm with two of my cousins. I would have found it more enjoyable to sway in a hammock with a book, looking up at leaves quivering in the liquidambar tree above, but the discomfort of displeasing my parents, who wanted me to socialise, outweighed my fear of moving among strangers.

My mother and I decided I should put on the pretty, drop-waist cream frock I'd worn a year before to the Year Six social. My aunt picked me up with her daughters and dropped us at the party, about an hour's drive away.

Beneath the bright lights of the shed, the usual discomfort I experienced around people became excruciating. The dress, which was soft and delicate, looked old-fashioned among everyone's jeans and checked shirts. I bobbed awkwardly, trying to dance. My cousins went off to chat to people they knew, but I had no idea of how to conduct a conversation. Bored and miserable, I ended up in a plastic chair near the fence, trying to ignore the girl next to me sitting in a boy's lap, kissing him with slurping noises that were loud enough for me to hear.

When the night finally ended and my aunt dropped me off in the driveway, my mother was waiting up. She'd switched on the verandah light so I could find my way indoors.

'How was it?' she asked as I opened the screen door.

'Terrible.' I went to my room.

Like Campbell Praed with Maud, she wanted me to have a lovely time at the ball.

As I grew into my late teens, I became increasingly anxious that I didn't have a boyfriend. I was raised in a conservative rural community and most of the adults I knew were married. Divorce wasn't common, let alone homosexuality. Observing the people around me, it seemed to me that, to be acceptable, a woman needed to get married and have children. As a thirteen-year-old girl, I felt that my inability to interact well enough to find a boyfriend, or to be attractive enough to catch someone's eyes, made me a failure.

My parents or relatives sometimes casually asked, 'Do you have a boyfriend, Jess?'

These questions reminded me that I had a disability and that I wasn't like everyone else. Their unfairness stung: how could my family expect me to find a boyfriend when I couldn't even hold a simple conversation, let alone understand the rules for dating?

At the end of my final year at primary school, the graduating students and their parents gathered for a social at the Boggabri RSL, the one at which I first wore that drop-waist frock. Large, round circles of coloured cardboard were pinned to the curtains. Written on them were phrases describing each of the children. 'Wired for Sound', mine read, a reference to my hearing aid and the frequency-modulation system I used to hear my teacher.

When the lights dimmed and music played, we were expected to dance. A boy who travelled with me on the bus to school asked me onto the floor. I swung my arms awkwardly. At the song's close, he attempted to lift me, as though I were a bride to be carried over a threshold. I was too heavy and fell from his arms onto the floor.

I wanted to weep. I was socially inept, so heavy I couldn't be lifted, and I was lying on a floor surrounded by my classmates and parents, all of them in stitches. Instead I stood, smiling, and pretended it was hilarious.

A year later, in my first year of high school, Oliver and I were invited to play at a music workshop at the other high school in town. We were both learning flute, and I liked its clear, high sound. This was the year I had the all-consuming crush on the golden-skinned boy. As I fitted my flute together, I saw him at the other end of the row of musicians and my heart began to hammer. Each glimpse of him throughout the day was like a sugar rush. In the afternoon, Mum came to the hall to pick us up. I packed up my flute and found her chatting to the boy's mother, whom she knew. I listened idly, until the boy approached. I began sweating and soon I couldn't take my eyes off the perfect symmetry of his face. After a few minutes, he wandered off.

In the car on the way home, Mum asked, 'Why were you looking at him like that?'

'Like what?'

'With such a soppy look on your face. It was embarrassing.'

I flushed and looked out the window, refusing to answer.

'Mum,' Oliver said from the back seat.

'Yes, dear?'

'Jess and I ate lunch on the seats under the tree, where everyone's schoolbags were. This dog came up and sniffed the bags, then it lifted its leg and pissed on one of them.'

I couldn't help myself; I started to laugh. A second later I resolved that, if my parents ever asked about boyfriends again, I would tell them to fuck off. From then on, to stop them asking questions when they delved into my private life, I would snap, 'It's none of your business.'

I kept writing, pouring my worries into characters and themes. At sixteen, inspired by the sunsets and dust of the film *Out of Africa*, and drawing on my hazy sense of the ostracism caused by racism (which was not very acute at this stage because I never listened to the news; that required concentration to hear), I wrote a story set in Africa about a young man who had been banished because he was disfigured. Despite his isolation, a young girl sought him out and came to love him. This was the first expression of what was to become the core of my work: the absolute redemption of a love that absolved the awkwardness and anxiety of being out of place.

A year later, I picked up Keri Hulme's *The Bone People*. I was fascinated by the poetry of Hulme's phrasing, and I liked the cleverness of her mute character, how his irrepressible nature shone through despite the flaws of the adults who were meant to take care of him. They were people who tried to be good but failed repeatedly. I identified with that.

Inspired, once more, by the dust of Blixen's work and the music of Hulme's, I wrote a ten-thousand-word story over two days. In it, a brother and a sister land on a dusty planet to attend a prestigious music school. They form complicated relationships with two rival music teachers, an internecine arrangement that climaxes with a death in the desert.

Reading this story now, saved in a file of my early writing, I'm surprised by its confidence. The style and dialogue are overblown and melodramatic, but a careful, steady tension rises from the sound plotting.

I'm reminded of my father, who would listen to my piano practice as he watched television in the next room. If I made a mistake, he'd shout, 'Wrong note!'

'Shut up!' I would yell back, irritated. I didn't have an ear for music because I was too deaf, although by the time I gave up learning the instrument, after eight years of lessons, I was beginning to hear when I played something wrong.

Although I didn't have my father's instinctive sense for when something was out of place in music, I did have it for writing. I can see that even at age seventeen, when I wrote this story, I had an intuition for how to put elements together in a story so that they harmonise.

A few years before this, I was fifteen, cast adrift from the comfort of the farm, which we had just left. I lay awake at night, fretting about my podginess, lack of social skills, and alienation because of my deafness. I thought about my godmother, a big-hearted woman who had been a hairdresser before she married and moved to her husband's property, a thirty-minute drive away from ours. She had an artificial eye, replacing the one she'd lost when she fell off a rocking horse when she was a child. Coincidentally, her husband also lost one of his eyes later in a farming accident.

When I had the respiratory arrest with meningitis, my godmother was at my bedside, praying. Every Christmas, she sent me beautiful gifts and picture books, many of them about God. When I stayed with her one weekend, she took me and her sons canoeing on a waterway on her property. Tall cliffs of pale-orange rock rose on either side of us. The water was tranquil, the air still, the sunlight mild. Christianity became bound with my godmother, the quietness of that afternoon, her gifts and enfolding hugs.

Sitting cross-legged on my bedroom floor and looking through the Bible and other books she sent me, I thought that God might be able to make me hear again and miraculously restore me to normalcy. I pored over accounts of Jesus healing the sick in the New Testament, and beseeched God nightly to return my hearing. No miracles manifested, however, and I remained deaf.

A few weeks before I left for university, I couldn't sleep again. I stared at the slats of my brother's bed above me. School in Armidale had been a relatively safe, if dull, haven and I was anxious about how to negotiate the new terrain of university, and how I would explain to everyone that I was deaf. The magnitude of it seemed enormous.

The next day, I found the phone number of a clairvoyant in my mother's *Woman's Day*.

The woman's voice at the end of the line was soft and gentle. She asked for my name, then said, 'How may I help you today, Jessica?'

'Uhm, I'm deaf,' I stammered. 'And what I want to know is... if...I'm ever going to be able to hear again.'

There was a pause, then the clairvoyant answered slowly, 'Well, Jessica, people don't always hear with their ears, they can hear in other ways. And I'm seeing something else here...writing? Do you write?'

I was startled. How had she worked that out? 'Yes, I've got a scholarship to start at uni next year, studying creative writing.' Blindsided, I put the phone down.

She hadn't answered my question, nor, deep down, had I expected her to. Yet she had recognised something powerful about me: that writing was integral to my identity and, therefore, to my deafness.

~

At the State Library of Queensland, I put the letters from Maud's brothers aside and turn to the mass of Rosa's writing. Unsure where to go next, I return to the first box in her archive, which contains proofs and manuscripts relating to her novels *Nyria* and *Soul of Nyria*, published in 1904 and 1931 respectively.

When Rosa moved to London in 1876, she stepped into a world that was entranced with the possibility of life beyond death. Darwinism had shaken many people's belief in a Christian god, but rather than leading to atheism it prompted a mushrooming of beliefs in spiritualism, theosophy, Rosicrucianism, palmistry and astrology.[46] This spiritual culture was a boon to Rosa, who had been interested in religion and the otherworldly since she was young.

The obsession with spirits was prompted by new and exciting inventions such as the telephone, telegraph and cinema. If one could hear a disembodied voice on the telephone, for example, or receive a message via telegraph, it seemed logical that one might hear the dead from a distance as well.[47] Rosa was captivated by these analogies. In a letter written in her later years, she raised the notion of 'a sort of "Talking Film" region in space where everything that ever has been is preserved'.[48] She believed that this region could be accessed as long as one had the right medium, tools or techniques. She called it the 'Memory of the Great Whole', an idea borrowed from theosophy.

The founders of the theosophical movement, Helena Blavatsky and Henry Steel Olcott, moved their headquarters from New York to India in 1875, settling on an estate outside Madras (now Chennai). In 1880, they stayed at the summer house of Alfred Percy Sinnett, an English journalist living in Simla (now Shimla), where he edited an English daily, *The Pioneer.* Sinnett was so enthusiastic in his support for theosophists that he didn't report properly on other affairs, and was sacked. In 1884 he returned to England and became president of the London Lodge of the Theosophical Society.

Theosophy, an offshoot of spiritualism, revolves around the idea of reincarnation, or that what happened in an individual's life is determined by their actions in previous lives. For Rosa, its tenet of reincarnation helped to explain the tragedies of her current life, including her difficult relationship with her husband and her daughter's deafness.

As she became increasingly famous through her writing, Rosa gained access to renowned literary and spiritualist circles. Soon she counted Blavatsky and Olcott among her acquaintances, and hosted a salon for them in her Talbot Square house. She also came to know Alfred Sinnett, and invited him to contribute an essay to *For Their Sakes*, the volume she edited to raise money for Maud's school. Other contributors to the book included Justin McCarthy, an author and Irish Nationalist Member of Parliament, who became a close friend and literary collaborator; the playwright and poet Herman Charles Merivale, who took Maud to pantomimes; and the feminist artist Louise Jopling. While these celebrities charmed Rosa and enriched her life, it was the connection with Alfred Sinnett that was to change her and Maud's lives completely.

~

'I think we missed the turn-off!' The street directory was open in my lap. Mum and I were at the lights on a main road on the North Shore of Sydney. I was seventeen. Mum hated driving in Sydney and I was sure she'd yell at me the way Dad yelled at her when she didn't read the map properly.

'It doesn't matter, we'll work it out.' Her tone was calm.

We reached a low-roofed brick house in a leafy cul-de-sac. Mum switched off the ignition. 'The man will run you through some tests, then in a few days we'll come back and he'll talk to you about what you're good at.'

'What sort of tests?'

'I don't know. He'll explain them to you.'

'Will you be with me?'

'No, I'll wait here in the car.'

'What will you do?'

'I have a magazine.'

I was nervous about being left on my own, even though the man, middle-aged with thinning hair, seemed mild and unthreatening. He took me into a room with a desk.

'They're logic and patterning tests. You need to listen to the tape recorder and write your answers in this book. I have a client in the room next door, but if you need help, just press the intercom button here.' He pointed to a button on the desk.

I nodded. The tests were straightforward, but for one section I couldn't hear clearly. I contemplated the black, square intercom button, weighing up the anxiety of trying to hear the man's voice, which would be obscured by crackling. If I couldn't hear, he'd have to leave his client and come into the room to help me. I couldn't bear the thought of making such a fuss. Instead I rewound and played the tape until I made out the words.

When I came out, my mother was waiting with the careers adviser.

'I noticed you didn't use the intercom,' he said.

'Oh no,' Mum laughed. 'Jessica would never do that. She likes to work things out on her own.'

We returned a few days later, this time with Dad, and the man explained the results of the assessments to us. 'Your deafness causes you a great deal of frustration, and you need to express this in creative ways. I suggest you do creative writing at the University of Wollongong.'

As Dad drove the car out of the cul-de-sac, I opened a catalogue the careers adviser gave us containing the course description. I had never once thought about the links between creating a book and the finished product that I had studied for English at school, or read avidly on car trips. I could take this delight I had, of making worlds and connections, and do it *all day*. This, I thought as I read the small, compact print, was exactly what I wanted to do.

A few months later, I included my story set in the desert in an application to study creative writing at the University of Wollongong. In early summer, Dad drove Mum and me the seven hours to the university for an interview.

The creative arts building was still being built, so I sat for the interview in a demountable. My story lay on the table before three interviewers, all of whom were men.

'This is a good piece of work,' one of them said.

'I wrote it in a weekend. It just flowed out.'

The men nodded.

I can't recall any other details, except the room full of young people waiting outside. It was the mid-1990s and they wore jeans and flannel shirts, even though they weren't country people. I was unnerved by their lack of familiarity; they seemed menacing.

I was accepted into the course. Mum organised my accommodation at college and arranged for the Creative Arts faculty's year adviser to help me choose my subjects. She explained how to open a bank account and bought me new clothes and rechargeable batteries for my FM system. My Tertiary Entrance Rank meant I was eligible for a faculty scholarship, and she took care of that, too.

'I spoke to the people at the university and they said the lady who runs the college is very nice. She'll look after you if you have any problems,' she explained as we left home.

I nodded.

Mum and I drove to Sydney and stayed with my sister, then living in Waverton around the corner from the apartment in which our parents had met. The harbour spread beneath us, its sheen like slate. The next day we drove to Wollongong. After installing me in my room at the college, my sister later told me, she and Mum went back to the car and burst into tears.

I didn't cry and I wasn't particularly homesick, although I must have been overwhelmed because, unusually, I fell asleep immediately every night. What did distress me were the buildings full of strangers. In the dining hall, I sensed I was expected to sit near someone and have a conversation, as people usually did over meals. But I didn't know how to begin. I felt like I was drowning.

Unable to bear this ordeal more than once a day, I stopped going to breakfast, arriving just in time to make myself a sandwich for lunch at the bar at the back of the meal hall. On the weekends there was no sandwich bar, so we needed to find lunch for ourselves. This involved going to the shops in town. As I had never caught a bus other than to school, and as I was reluctant to have a humiliating conversation with a bus driver I might not be able to hear, I walked to the nearby corner store and bought an ice cream for lunch.

At lunchtime on the campus, I would search for a piece of lawn free of duckshit and unwrap my sandwich, my first meal for the day. I was so nauseous with stress that I could usually only eat half of it. In six weeks I lost six kilos, and my jeans hung from my hipbones. But on the grass I'd open my copy of Aritha van Herk's *Judith* for my English course on women writers, and my mind caught fire.

It was the same with my writing classes. My first teacher, back in the demountables, was a poet, Deb Westbury. 'Write for at least ten minutes every day,' she told us. 'Don't stop to edit, because it doesn't matter how bad it is. Just write.'

I bought a journal, the first of many that would fill my bookcases. In my small room in the college, stars burning beyond the tall window, I scribbled on page after page into the hours after midnight. My writing in this journal was terrible, but uninhibited. I wrote about sitting alone in my English classes, conversations and laughter bubbling around me while I slowly drew out my notepad. I would sit quietly, my shoulders hunched and my hands clasped in my lap, but when the lecturer walked in, I straightened my spine.

The room swelled with the promise of ideas, writers and stories.

I also described how, during the college's orientation week, we'd had to draw the name of an orientation leader from a hat and then buy them a drink on an excursion to the pub. I had no idea what to do, or even of what people drank, as I'd never been inside a pub before.

As we walked through the pub's doors, I alighted on a solution. I approached the girl whose name was written on the small scrap of paper in my hand.

'Hi, Anna, I owe you a drink. What would you like?'

'A rum and coke.'

'Okay, got it.'

I went to the bar and ordered her drink but, not knowing what to drink myself, I left shortly afterwards.

If my mind blanked as I wrote in my journal, thinking of the next thing to say, I didn't stop. I wrote, *keep writing keep writing keep writing*.

The next semester, my teacher was John Scott. A clever, lugubrious man, he mused in his ironic way, 'If I practised writing as much as a footballer trained, I'd be a champion by now.' So I continued with my mad, furious, awful writing over the summer. When I returned the following year and the class workshopped a short story I'd written, John Scott asked with a small smile, 'Have you been drinking?'

'No! I've been writing.'

As I look at the pattern of Rosa's life, it's evident that she became a writer not only through grit and determination, but also through her skilful use of networks. Through her husband's family she met her first publishers, Chapman and Hall, and through Frederick Sartoris, her neighbour at Rushden, she met politician Justin McCarthy. She collaborated with McCarthy on a number of works, including *The Grey River* (1889), illustrated by Maud's art teacher Mortimer Menpes. Rosa's books gave her an introduction to celebrities such as Oscar Wilde, whom she fictionalised in her novel *Affinities*. In a sheaf of paper in her archives titled 'Phrases of the Eighties', she typed up one of Wilde's aphorisms,'I love superstition.The Reformation killed our superstition, & so it killed our art', and later used it in her novel *The Scourge-Stick* (1898).[49] She also encountered Rudyard Kipling at a dinner organised by her publisher Frederic Chapman, of Chapman & Hall, describing him as 'a young man of about twenty three with a black moustache, keen eyes, & frank unconventional manner', who spoke at times 'with all the cynicism of three & twenty & an experience of social life at Simla'.[50] Rosa was in the thick of London's artistic society, and she loved it.

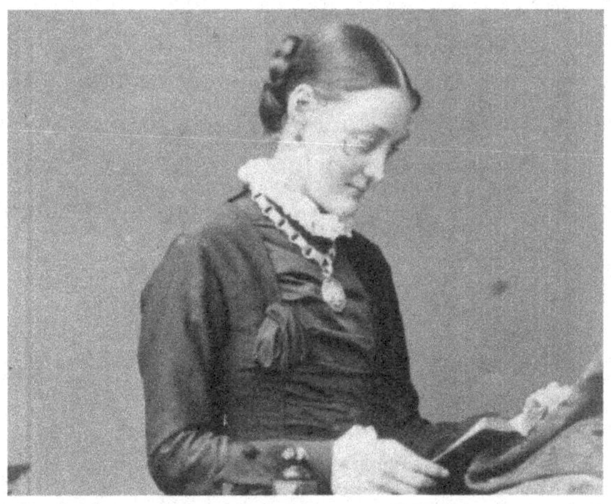

Rosa Praed. John Oxley Library,
State Library of Queensland, Neg No: 66725

I feel some envy of Rosa's networking in literary circles, especially when I contrast it with my first year as a writer at Wollongong, when I was completely alone. I studied and wrote constantly because I had no friends with whom to hang out. When I tired of writing, I walked to the lighthouse on the headland between the city's beaches. The tough, closely cropped grass, stark white pillar of the lighthouse and relentless ocean mirrored my loneliness. I watched tourists and families with their children taking photos of one another, the wind blowing my hair into my face.

In my second year in the residential college I made a friend who was also studying creative writing. During the week she wrestled with the temperamental VCR in the games room until it worked. We watched French films, which I liked because they had subtitles and I didn't need to strain to hear the film. But she went home to Sydney on weekends to her family and part-time job in a bookstore. Lonely once more, I walked the still, quiet streets of Wollongong. The escarpment, that great shelf of forest, rose behind the city like a green prison. It wasn't until I made the great leap to Berkeley two years later that my life opened up like a sunflower, bright yellow and bristling with black seeds of possibility.

Was this what it was like for Rosa, I think in the State Library as I leaf through her typed account of meeting medium Nancy Harward? Did things suddenly, for the first time in her life, feel *right*?

~

After her trip with Maud around the world, Rosa returned to England in 1895 to find Campbell had run out of money. He was relying on cheques from his brother and had moved into a flat on his own. Although his relationship with Rosa had broken down, he remained very attached to his children. Maud wrote to her aunt Dorothy and explained that Campbell, very unwell with pneumonia and recovering from a hunting accident, 'is still in his bachelor flat and comes to see us nearly every day'.[51]

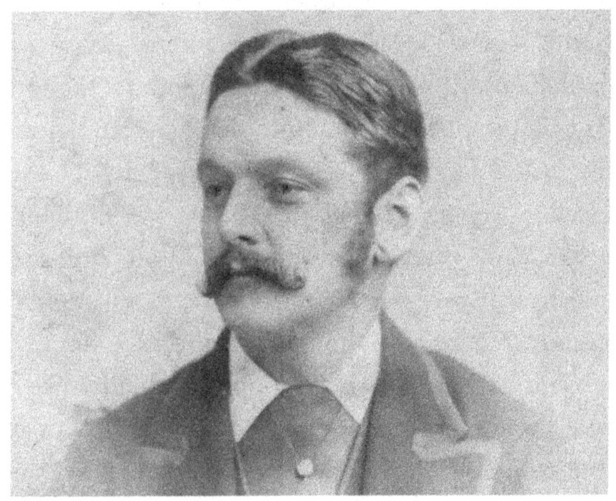

Campbell Praed. John Oxley Library, State Library of Queensland, Neg No: 197572

Four years later, in 1899, the marriage was over. Rosa's eldest son Bulkley, then twenty-four, discussed the implications of a separation from Campbell. He pointed out to Rosa that 'you must have thoroughly realised that you can do nothing for him from any beneficial point of view. The idea of providing a home which can be of any use to him borders on the ridiculous.'[52] By this point, Rosa and Campbell were not on speaking terms. Bulkley, who had lunched with his father, wrote to his mother, 'Father said that he had not heard from you for some time, whereupon I made the same retort on your behalf.'[53]

In Rosa's novels, the theme of an incompatible couple trapped in an unhappy marriage is a frequent motif, appearing explicitly in *The Bond of Wedlock* (1887). Her protagonist Harvey becomes depraved through his loveless marriage, in which his wife, Ariana, 'had always, from the day of her betrothal, shrunk from her husband's rough caresses. Her marriage had seemed a degradation.'[54] Harvey's physical abuse and desertion of Ariana, while simultaneously having an affair, points to the decay of a society that will not allow women to divorce even if a man 'were to beat [his wife] black and blue all over every day for a month'.[55] It is a bleak novel, suggesting that Rosa was troubled by her marriage for many years before her separation. Still, she refused to countenance divorce on account of the social stigma and the precariousness of her and Campbell's finances.

In the late 1890s, Rosa's theosophist friend Alfred Sinnett introduced her to the writer and doctor Arthur Conan Doyle. Rosa came to know Doyle and his wife 'intimately', and found them people of 'keen intellect, wide-reading and the doctor, especially, of a scientific bent'.[56] Doyle had established a practice in Portsmouth in 1882, and one of his patients, Lieutenant General Thomas Harward, became a friend. Harward, previously stationed in India, had been a gunnery officer in the relief of Lucknow, during the 1857 mutiny of Indian soldiers in the East India Company's Bengal Presidency Army. His daughter Nancy was born in Agra in 1864 and was sent to England at age three. When her father retired from the army in Portsmouth, Nancy acted in plays with him and Doyle at 'Kingston Lodge', the Harwards' home. A program for 'Amateur Theatricals' dated 10 August 1886 lies in Rosa's archives at the John Oxley Library. The cast of seven included Arthur Conan Doyle, Nancy and her father.[57]

Nancy and her father also practised table-rapping sessions with the Doyles, during which they hoped to make çontact with spirits. According to Doyle's account in his notebook, they placed their hands on the table, pushed at it until there was enough motion, and recited the alphabet. The table responded with a rap at specific letters, which eventually formed into words, including the phrase, 'I have not nor ever shall forget you, darling little Nancy. Please love mother for my sake. Henry Hastie.'[58] Henry was Nancy's cousin, who had died three years before. With this revelation, the temperature plummeted and, Doyle wrote, 'Miss Harward became icy cold and experienced a sensation as of soft hands patting her upon the palm with a strong feeling that someone was standing behind her. At the command of the spirits, we discontinued the sitting.'[59]

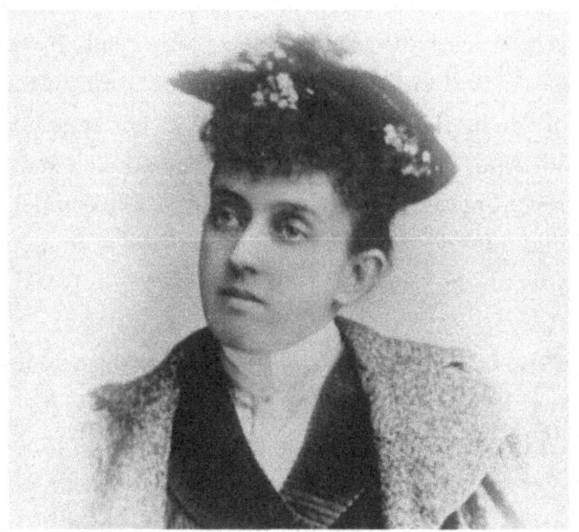

Nancy Harward. John Oxley Library, State Library of Queensland, Neg No: 114482

Nancy also had the ability to fall into a trance and speak as a German princess, captured and enslaved in ancient Rome. The Doyles described her psychic abilities to Rosa, adding that Nancy wanted to move to London to further her writing career. Nancy had published some stories, and received encouragement from Doyle. Intrigued, Rosa began a correspondence with Nancy, then invited her to London to meet.

Among the first sheaves of paper in the first box of Rosa's archives in the John Oxley Library lies a typed account of this meeting. It opens, 'This is how I made the acquaintance of Nyria, slave attendant upon Julia the daughter of Titus, emperor of Rome, 79–81 AD.'[60] The attraction between the two women at their first meeting was immediate:

> A sudden mutual sympathy sprang up between us. I was struck by the quiet charm of her talk, by her candour and, curiously, by her common sense. More than all, by the look of spirituality in her large grey eyes. And some quality in her, behind her gentle reserve, appealed to me in an indescribable manner. I could not tell what the quality was – it had strength, purity, abidingness.[61]

The words *sudden*, *struck*, *appealed* suggest that this meeting was a case of love at first sight. Meanwhile, Nancy wrote in her diary, 'I met Mrs Praed at Chichester on about the 20th October [1899]. On Sunday the 5th Nov I spent the afternoon with W. & then supped for the last time in the old way at St Swithins. Monday the 6th I went to Elm Park Gardens', where Rosa lived.[62] That Nancy ate 'for the last time in the old way' indicates that her move to

London was not just a visit, but something more permanent. In little more than two weeks, Rosa and Nancy founded a relationship that was to last another thirty years.

For a few years, before things starting going badly wrong in Rosa's family, she must have been extraordinarily happy. Her biographer Patricia Clarke refers to Lillian Faderman's *Surpassing the Love of Men* to explain Rosa's relationship with Nancy. Faderman argues that intense friendships between women were largely asexual and 'were love relationships in every sense except perhaps the genital'.[63] Clarke adds that, while Rosa and Nancy's friendship was intense, Rosa 'found Radclyffe Hall's lesbian novel *The Well of Loneliness* "nauseating"'; it seemed 'to attack & try to make impossible the purest friendship between women, of which there are so many cases'.[64] Meanwhile, queer studies scholar Damien Barlow rightly observes that heterosexual readings of Rosa have sidelined Nancy, reducing her to 'a ghostly eccentricity in Praed's life and work, a queer spectre adding peculiarity to the margins'.[65] He bases his analysis, however, on Colin Roderick's odd 1948 biography of Rosa, *In Mortal Bondage: The Strange Life of Rosa Praed*, which borders on fiction at times and casts Nancy in the role of slave girl, borrowing from her Roman incarnation. While theirs was at times an unequal relationship, with Rosa stymieing Nancy's literary career and appropriating her material, it was undeniably deep, reciprocal and abiding. As I read Rosa's notes on *Nyria*, which she wrote in collaboration with Nancy, it becomes clear that their relationship was much more than a friendship.

The novel *Nyria* opens on a street at the foot of the Palatine Hill in Rome. Valeria, a noblewoman, is carried along in a litter and one of her slaves clears the way with his stave. He hits a young girl, Nyria, and knocks her over. When Valeria chastises the slave, Nyria is instantly besotted: 'At the sound of Valeria's voice she had reddened and then gone pale' while her eyes, 'large, soft, appealing, and suffused with tears gave [Valeria] an adoring look'.[66] Such is Nyria's devotion that, when Nyria's owner dies, Nyria begs to be bought by Valeria. She becomes a Christian, then an unlawful sect in Rome, and acts as an intermediary between Valeria and her lover Lucianus. When that relationship fails, Valeria, in her distress, unwittingly reveals where Nyria and the Christians worship. Nyria is captured and fed to the lions, becoming a martyr for refusing to give up her faith.

There are moments of unmistakeable tenderness between the women, beginning with the initial, highly charged meeting between Valeria and Nyria. Valeria is as affected as Nyria, finding herself 'strangely stirred'.[67] Stephanus, a shop owner who is enamoured of Nyria, comments on her adoration of Valeria: 'Thou art indeed bewitched!'[68] The instantaneous attraction mirrors Rosa's account of her meeting with Nancy in her transcripts in the archives: 'A sudden mutual sympathy sprang up between us.'[69] Eventually, Rosa came to believe that she was the current incarnation of Valeria, as Nancy was of Nyria. If their ghosts had appeared in the past and the present, then it meant they would reincarnate as a couple in the future and that they would be together forever.

In *The Apparitional Lesbian*, scholar Terry Castle describes how lesbians and their desire have been described in literature as 'ghostly' so that they can be exorcised. Castle writes, 'Given the threat that sexual love between women inevitably poses to the workings of patriarchal arrangement, it has often been felt necessary to deny the carnal *bravada* of lesbian existence. The hoary misogynist challenge, "But what do lesbians do?" insinuates as much: *This cannot be. There is no place for this.*'[70] They are rendered, as Castle shows through numerous examples, as ghostly.

If lesbianism is equated with ghosts, and if Rosa coded her relationship with Nancy in relation to spirits from the start, then there is overwhelming evidence that theirs was a lesbian relationship.

Perhaps Rosa felt something settling into place when Nancy moved into her house, the way I did when I walked down Sproul Plaza at Berkeley, reassured by a sense of finally fitting in. I loved sitting in cafés reading or studying until eleven o'clock at night; the hard, clear light of mornings that stretched into a flawless blue sky; people drumming on plastic buckets in the evening at the university's plaza; Telegraph Avenue cluttered with tarot-card readers sitting at tables at the intersections, and bearded men selling silver jewellery. For a white girl from country New South Wales, it was a revelation to walk down the street and find myself in the minority.

I was taught by writers such as Clark Blaise and Robert Hass, went to lectures by Judith Butler, saw (but didn't hear, because there were no hearing facilities in the hall) the poet Seamus Heaney, and went to the launch of a journal that had published some of my poems, although I felt so ill-at-ease in the small room of people that I left after half an hour. I met some students from Australia and travelled with them to Yosemite National Park, awed by its grandeur. I spent Christmas in Rochester, New York, with more Australian friends, then caught a train down to Chicago with a blanket my host had kindly given me because I had the flu. From Chicago I caught an Amtrak train from east to west across the country, stopping off at Denver for the last night of the twentieth century.

Somehow I got talking to a boy on the train. He seemed my age and was my height, with mousy hair. I found he was staying at the same youth hostel as me. The hostel owner had offered to pick me up when I called from the station, but when I located a payphone and dialled the number for the hostel, I couldn't hear where he told me to meet him. I decided to head outside and hope for the best.

The boy followed me to the kerb. 'Can I share a room with you? It'd be cheaper that way.'

I didn't reply, trying to work out where the owner might see me. After ten minutes, there was no sign of anyone looking to pick us up.

'Is this the right spot?' the boy asked.

'I don't know.'

'You don't know?' he jeered.

'I'm deaf. I couldn't hear him very well on the phone.'

The boy blanched and stammered an apology, but I ignored him and moved towards the station's entrance. I noticed a middle-aged man in a station wagon who looked like he was waiting, and introduced myself. It was the right person, so we climbed into the car.

When we reached the hostel, I said to the boy, 'I don't need to share a room with you. I've made my own booking.'

'But I've got a girlfriend.'

I shrugged. He had been rude to me and it wasn't my problem that he hadn't got himself organised.

I spent the last night of the twentieth century watching celebrations around the world on television, too sick from the flu to go out.

The next day the hostel owner, a kind man with a bad cut of greying hair, drove me to the Natural History Museum. Entry was free because it was the first day of a new century. I looked at the taxidermied animals of the American savannah and ate my sandwich by a lake after pacing to find a section free of duckshit. A few hours later, as we agreed, the hostel owner picked me up. I wonder, now, if he had overheard my conversation with the boy when we got out of the car. I was twenty-one but looked younger, and I am short. I must have seemed very small and naïve. No wonder my mother had cried at the airport.

On 2 January, he dropped me back at the train station. After another overnighter on Amtrak, I woke up and watched snowy trees drifting past. It was my twenty-second birthday and I was finally growing up.

When I returned to Australia a month later, energised and confident, I couldn't bear to stay in the quietness of Wollongong any longer. I moved into an apartment in Surry Hills with two friends of Oliver's and commuted to Wollongong to finish my Honours degree, which I divided between an analysis of nineteenth-century botanist Georgiana Molloy's letters in the English Department, and writing a poetry sequence under Alan Wearne's supervision in the Creative Writing Department. I was happy to be around Oliver again and I adored his friends, who quickly became mine. We watched *Video Smash Hits* on Saturday mornings, picnicked at Darling Harbour for the opening of the Sydney Olympics, and walked across the Sydney Harbour Bridge for reconciliation on a bitter winter's day. The air, though cold, was full of hope.

In between writing and commuting, I began temping a few days a week to save money. As I tried to work out what to do when I finished my degree, my thoughts often turned to my father and his art.

On the farm, Dad fed his pigs first thing in the morning, then worked with his brothers and father at their combined piggery. After that they ploughed paddocks, sowed grain, harvested, crutched sheep, docked lambs, and rounded up and branded cattle. When the day's work was done, Dad painted watercolours in his studio, a separate building from the house that he'd built himself. Shaped like a ship, it stood on thick, sturdy trunks. Out the front was a brick patio, on which Mum placed large pots of cumquat trees. Before this, Dad had painted in the laundry, surrounded by his work tools, his rifle and the washing machine.

Dad's work reflected the taste of the people among whom we lived, for his patrons were local. He painted paddocks and gum trees; views of gardens from large glass windows; cows, sheep and spinifex; flower arrangements on checked tablecloths; country pubs and dusty roads. He also travelled, then held exhibitions of places he'd been to: India, Egypt, Italy, Greece, Russia and Mongolia.

After dinner, Oliver and I would traipse across the lawn to the studio, dew and grass clippings sticking to our ugg boots. We sat on the rough, camel-hair carpet Mum and Dad had bought in India, and drew cartoons on offcuts of cardboard that Dad used for mounts. Dad whistled or hummed along to musicals on the stereo. Sometimes I stood beside him, my head just reaching above his desk, watching his brush stain the paper with pigment.

Mum had bought me a sketchbook, and on weekends I sat at the table on the verandah with the view of low hills, practising my drawing. Sometimes Dad stood over my shoulder, watching. Ever frugal, he complained to Mum, 'She's wasting good paper.'

For once, I happened to overhear and retorted, 'How else am I supposed to get better at drawing?'

I deliberately turned to a new page and drew large, extravagant shapes across it.

When visitors came for morning tea, gathering around the round wooden table in the dining room that we children had stippled with our pencils, I laid my sketchbook on the table and turned the pages for them.

'Very good, Jess,' they murmured over cups of tea in my mother's blue-and-white Figgjo Lotte china from Norway.

When I was seven, I copied an image from one of my picture books, a black swan gliding on dark water in the shadow of an overhanging tree. I coloured it in with a watery set of paints Mum picked up from Kmart. She entered it in the junior section at the local art show.

We drove into town to look at the show, held in the Boggabri RSL. The walls were hung with hessian, to which the paintings were pinned. Dad's paintings were in the main section. I wandered into the children's section in a separate room. As I drew closer, I spotted my painting, a blue rosette pinned beside it. I fingered the folds of ribbon with a smile, happiness crackling inside me.

Watching Dad paint at night and listening to him talk about art ('Sometimes you just have to paint what people want to make money') helped me to understand how I could make a living from writing and create something of which I was proud. More than this, I realised, the process of writing was crucial to my wellbeing. Through it I expressed my awkwardness around people, the pricks of humiliation I felt at not being able to move seamlessly through interactions, and the enduring loneliness that, I assumed, would never leave me.

And of course, there was the pleasure of writing: the delight of capturing the drunken flight of a swallowtail butterfly; learning the symbolism of characters' names; the puzzle of fitting together plot and structure in a satisfying way; the relief, after teeth-grinding effort, of finding a perfect cadence – a sentence or paragraph that concluded harmoniously – for an ending. There was the way I could transmute my moments of sadness into splendour, for writing was like taking the lid off a jar of once-tart, preserved apricots and finding they had become sweet.

I wanted to do nothing else but write; I just had to figure out a way to finance it.

When I completed my final year, my parents and Oliver drove to Wollongong for my graduation ceremony. Dad insisted we stay overnight at Thirroul in the motel in which Brett Whiteley had overdosed and died.

Alan Wearne met us in the hall where the ceremony took place, wearing his carpet slippers. He didn't stay for the ceremony, but he still wanted to meet my parents. Most years since I have left Wollongong, he has phoned to wish me a happy birthday.

I graduated with First Class Honours and a University Medal, a reward not only for the hours of loneliness and hard work, but also for the pleasures of writing in my cramped room. My marks were good enough to get me into a PhD course and I wanted to do more research in English literature, but I knew that if I started a doctorate, I would never write the novel that had been gathering, over the last few years, like sugars and proteins in a seed. I enrolled in a Master of Arts in Writing at the University of Technology, Sydney, and began the novel that would become *A Curious Intimacy*.

Inspired by the letters of Georgiana Molloy, the nineteenth-century botanist whose letters I had researched for Honours the year before, as well as by the story of Rachel Henning, who was happiest on horseback and sleeping beneath stars, and by my enduring love of romances such as *Jane Eyre*, I began to write a story of two nineteenth-century women who fell in love in the forests of south-west Western Australia. I was motivated, as of old, by my desire to find a form or shape that was beyond the mainstream. While I had read many stories of men and women falling in love in the bush, I hadn't encountered many lesbian romances in Australian literary fiction, which was odd given the prevalence of same-sex desire.

I knew that, historically, lesbians had felt compelled to hide their sexuality the way I hid my deafness, or to code it in ways that needed to be deciphered. It seemed to me that they also moved in a world that, arranged and controlled by the patriarchy, wasn't designed for their desires, the way I was trying to survive as a deaf woman in a hearing world.

When I began to write, though, the novel started with a woman who had lost her child and went mad with grief. This was a story that had been with me since I was born.

In between Bella and me was the boy named Hamish, whose grave stood at the back of my grandparents' house. In photos, he's a smiling, chubby baby, laughing when someone pokes him in the belly. When he was eight months old, he died in an accident. There was an inquest at the courthouse.

'It was just a formality,' Mum explained. She added that people would cross the road when they saw her in town.

I was horrified. It would have been hard enough on my parents without people avoiding them.

'They weren't being malicious. They didn't know what to say. It was easier to avoid me.'

In a small country town, where you know most people, crossing the road would have been unmistakeable.

The experience of ostracism resonated with me because I felt it strongly myself. At age eight I sat on the cement steps outside the classroom, waiting for the bus. At the park across the road was a birthday party with balloons and crepe-paper streamers. Every child in my class had been invited, except me. When the school bus arrived, I stepped through the doors alone and pulled out my book.

Children take their cues from adults. One Christmas the Anglican minister came to our classroom to direct the nativity play. I sat cross-legged on the new blue carpet, hoping I might get a role as Mary or an angel. Four other girls were picked, however, scrambling up into their places at the front of the room. Perhaps I might be a shepherd, then. There were more girls than boys in the class, so it would be okay for them to be shepherds. The minister picked out three shepherds and moved on to the animals. I could be a dog or a goat, I reasoned. I could practise barking or bleating at Oliver. Soon there was only me and a little boy who occasionally wet his pants, sitting on the floor. The other children ran through the script while we watched. After school, I described to my mother what had happened. She must have rung the minister, because the next day I was in the play.

My experiences of ostracism, and Mum's comment about people avoiding her at the point she needed them most, stayed with me. In *A Curious Intimacy*, the protagonist Ellyn finds her baby will not wake in the cot. She becomes deranged from grief, and her small town shuns her until Ingrid, a botanist, arrives on her doorstep. Ingrid falls for Ellyn, and in the generous sweep of her affection, Ellyn begins to recover and grow.

There it is again: a love that redeems all.

Looking at the sheaf of writing on Nyria and on Rosa's life with Nancy, in the well-lit room beside the Brisbane River, and returning from my thoughts on Rosa's romance and my writing, I wonder about the impact on Maud, who now had to share her mother's company. As a deaf person who read lips and bodies, Maud would have been sensitive to the interactions between Rosa and Nancy. Also, having spent her whole life with her mother, she would have been aware of changes in Rosa's behaviour.

Maud spent so much time with her mother that, in letters, she failed to separate their identities. She frequently took on Rosa's voice, or conflated it with her own. Writing to her grandfather from Potters Bar, thirty kilometres north of London, Maud complained of 'our present companion, as she talks and talks all the time, and makes such a fuss over a petty fault. In order to get rid of her, we are going to Cannes, and it may be a good excuse for her to go away. Mother and I feel quite sure that we should be happier if we are alone, and go about together.'[71] Maud might have found the companion tiring because concentrating on her voluble speech would have been exhausting, but her use of 'we', the adoption of her mother's feelings, and reference to the future they will spend together, shows how closely Maud aligned herself with Rosa.

In another letter to her grandfather written when she was seventeen, Maud commented, 'It is difficult to find a quiet meditation to keep away from the bustle of things. It would be delightful to lead a peaceful and sweet life like a nun in a convent, and have only a few friends in which we can trust confidence [sic] – but Father likes having a kind of frivolous life so we must please him.'[72] While Maud might have enjoyed life in a nunnery, where the lack of chatter would be a relief, the disapproving reference to her father's frivolity suggests that her mother's voice is firmly embedded in her own.

I can't help but think that Maud would have been jealous of Nancy, if my own feelings are anything to go by.

One morning in the Randwick apartment I shared with Oliver, I woke up, shuffled to the kitchen and set the stovetop coffee maker on the element.

A boy appeared in the doorway.

'Hello,' I said, holding a spoonful of coffee grains.

'Hi, I'm a friend of Oliver's.'

I realised this was his latest squeeze, and that I wouldn't be seeing much of my brother for a while. I smiled thinly. 'Would you like some coffee? I can make extra.'

'That would be great, thanks.' His smile was more generous than mine, his teeth very white.

When Rosa travelled abroad with Nancy the year after they met, Maud continued to live with Campbell at his place in Wellingborough. Either she or Rosa had decided they no longer wanted to be under the same roof. When discussing options for what to do about the family home if Rosa and Campbell separated, Bulkley wrote, 'You could always if necessary have [Maud and her companion] for a month or two with you,' suggesting that Rosa was not the first choice for accommodating Maud.[73]

What could Maud have been thinking as her family began to fracture? She was by this time a healthy woman of twenty-five. Her closeness to Rosa, underscored by their long trip to Australia, Asia and Canada, was now clouded by a broken marriage and her mother's relationship with another woman. Maud was intelligent, observant and aware of social expectations. She read her mother's novels, with their racy plots driven by desire and marriage, and she watched women her own age marry and have children. She would have wondered about her own prospects. When she was fourteen, she wrote in a letter to her grandmother, 'I am glad that I have no sisters but three brothers. Had I any sisters, they would annoy or quarrel with me, but I would rather have sister-in-laws [sic]. They will promise to stay near when they are old.'[74] Whether or not Maud was saying what was expected of her in this letter, or voicing these thoughts of her own volition, it seems she could not see a future that didn't have her family in it.

The year before this letter, at age thirteen, Maud returned from a holiday with her father and brothers at the seaside in Mablethorpe, Lincolnshire, while her mother had been in France and Switzerland. Maud wrote to her grandmother, 'I am very glad to stay at home with Mother and Father forever.'[75] To her aunts Meta and Dorothy, she said of Rosa's return, 'we welcome her, and were very glad to have her again as we were very tired of her absence'.[76] For Maud, family was everything.

In March 1899, when Rosa and Campbell were not on speaking terms but before Rosa had met Nancy, Maud was at Campbell's place in Wellingborough with her companion, Marion Tenniel. She was content there, as Bulkley commented to their mother, 'At present she is so satisfied with Wellingborough that Father is talking of the difficulty of getting her away for a few days during the Northampton races.'[77]

Maud was close to her father and he longed for her to be happy. In 1891, when the Praeds moved from London to the country for a slower pace of life, Maud had expressed her desire to accompany

Rosa to Cannes, but, she explained in a letter to her grandmother, 'Father does not like my leaving him.'[78]

On the evening of 3 November 1901, two years after Rosa's first meeting with Nancy, Maud was again at the house in Wellingborough, playing chess with Campbell. He had been unwell, but the next day he attended a board meeting in London. While he was there, Maud sent a letter to her brother Humphrey in California. A charming and jocular young man, Humphrey oversaw the picking, transportation and marketing of citrus fruit, a job that took him around the country to interview buyers and, he told Maud, 'expiate on the elegance of our Fruit'.[79] He bought ponies for playing polo, one of which he'd named 'Nyria' after Rosa's work-in-progress, although she was 'rather skittish for the character'.[80] In her letter to her brother, Maud described their father as 'so much better'.[81]

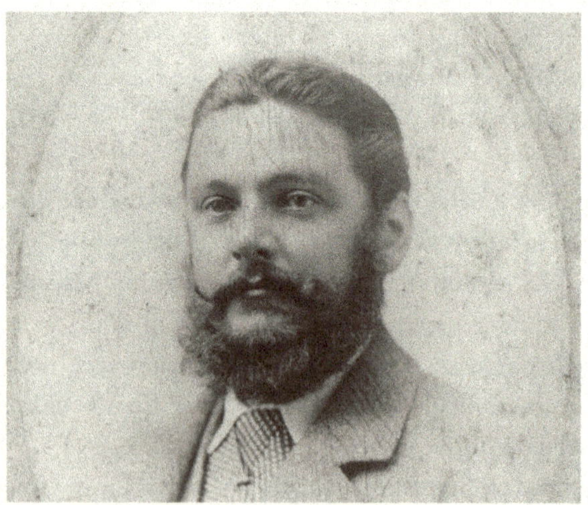

Humphrey Praed in San Francisco. John Oxley Library, State Library of Queensland, Neg No: 197577

After the board meeting, Campbell dined at his club, then walked through a thick fog to his chambers at Whitcomb Street on the Strand. When he reached his rooms on the first floor, where a man was waiting to see him, he began to cough violently. He said to his valet and the visitor, 'I believe I am dying.' The men tried to lay him upon a couch, but Campbell died in their arms. A doctor pronounced the cause of death a cerebral haemorrhage.[82]

Humphrey didn't learn of his father's death until a few weeks later, when he received a newspaper clipping from Maud. He wrote to Rosa immediately, expressing shock and concern for his mother and Maud. 'Poor Maud will be terribly grieved to lose him,' Humphrey wrote, then asked,

> What arrangements will be made about Maud & I call to mind a promise I made Father that Maud should never want for a friend whilst I was alive & now I want to say that if there is any difficulty about making suitable arrangements for Maud in England I will do my best to look after her out here. I shall not be able to do this very well out of my salary but if there is any provision made for her or the uncles would help, she can live with me and I will do my best to make her life a happy one.[83]

There seemed to be no longstanding provision for Maud to return to Rosa and Nancy.

At her father's funeral, Maud laid a wreath on his coffin with the inscription 'In loving memory of father'. She was described in the newspaper as 'his devoted daughter'.[84] Her distress over his loss was acute and persistent. In May 1902, she attempted a 'rest cure', then she was admitted to a nursing home. This did not soothe her, and ten months later Maud was sent to Holloway Sanatorium in Surrey, an asylum for middle-class patients suffering from insanity.[85] She'd had a breakdown.

~

In the light-filled John Oxley Library in Brisbane, I load the website for the National Archives in England. I often visited this glass-and-concrete building in Kew Gardens while I was in London, working on another research project for an Australian scholar. It contains more than eleven million historical government and public records, including the Domesday Book, photographs, posters, maps, drawings and paintings. In the catalogue's search box, I type 'Holloway Sanatorium'. The results page reveals that there are records held in an archive in Surrey.

It's time to go back to England.

I make a quick trip to New South Wales to say goodbye to my parents. My father hugs me so tightly that I feel like a little girl again. I bury my forehead into his shoulder and start to cry.

~

These days, as I cycle to the pool at Stones Corner, I try to imagine what would have happened if I hadn't met Maud and learned her story. Would I be here, chaining my bike to the rack and heading for the change rooms, if I hadn't heard her voice? What was it that drew me back to Brisbane after my research in the State Library? On the surface it was my sister who, wanting family to live nearby, constantly implored Oliver and me to return, but I wonder if it was something to do with Queensland, which had shaped Rosa in particular ways that had, in turn, shaped her daughter.

In the change rooms, I peel off my T-shirt and shorts and pull on my swimmers. I wrestle silicone into my good ear to protect it against infection and walk swiftly over the hot cement pavement to the water. The day is humid, waiting for the prick and gush of a storm. I pass Mango, the resident lorikeet. There's a sign on his cage warning people not to poke him because he'll nip, nor to feed him. A few weeks later he'll have a heart attack from too many Twisties. His replacement will be Blueberry, a baby lorikeet.

I lower myself into the water, pull on my goggles and kick off. With my ear stoppered up, I am completely deaf. I pull myself through kilometres of water, free to focus on the shifting shadows on the bottom of the pool, the rhythm of my breath and, when the storm breaks, the speckle of rain on my back.

Born one hundred and four years after Maud, I've learned that the attitudes to deafness that corralled her life still enclose mine. But there is a crucial difference: she helped me to recognise them, and to escape.

~

After saying goodbye to my parents, following my stints in the archives in Canberra and Brisbane, I fly back to England and arrange to visit the Surrey History Centre. It's a plain municipal building in Woking, some fifty kilometres south-west of London.

Over the nineteenth century, a booming population meant greater numbers of mentally ill people who needed care. More asylums were created to cater for them. In 1808 the County Asylums Act was passed to establish asylums for the poor and mentally ill, who were largely kept in jail. Progress in building the institutions was slow, however, so in 1845 the Lunacy Act and County Asylums Act were passed to establish a network of regulated public institutions.

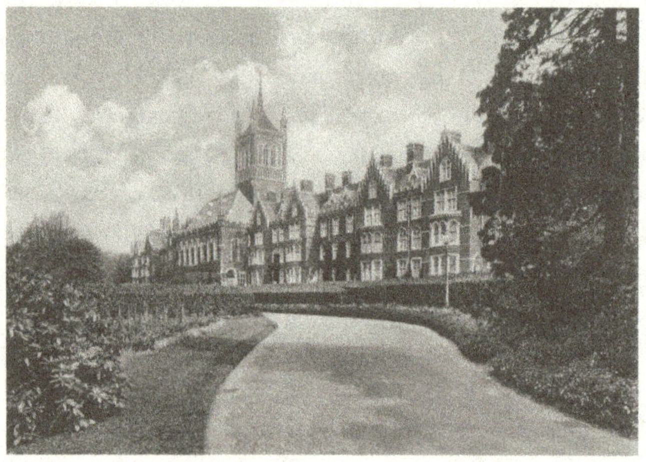

Holloway Sanatorium, view from the drive.
Surrey History Centre, 2620/6/26

The nineteenth century also saw the emergence of a middle class who thought it inappropriate for unwell family members to be incarcerated with paupers. They couldn't afford lengthy home care or a private hospital, but were too affluent for the pauper asylum.[86] Responding to this, Thomas Holloway, a wealthy philanthropist who made his fortune by patenting medicine, founded Holloway Sanatorium in 1885. According to the periodical *The Builder*, there were rules attached to admission, namely that 'no patient will be allowed to remain an inmate of the institution for a longer period than twelve months; no patient will be received whose case is considered hopeless; no patient will be allowed to enter the Sanatorium after having been once discharged'.[87]

The building was designed by architect Henry William Crossland in a Franco-Flemish style, and its grounds stretched over twenty-two acres of St Ann's Heath near Virginia Water, Surrey. With rolling lawns, cricket fields, gardens and private villas that could be rented by patients, their families and servants, it was designed to distract patients from their mental distress. Every inch of the walls were decorated because it was thought that plain walls were uncomfortable for mad people.[88]

In the History Centre in Woking, I'm directed to a cavernous room with windows looking onto a suburban street. I'm given a pair of gloves and a large leather-bound book. My pulse picks up as I carry it to a wide table and lift it carefully onto foam supports. I open the stiff cover and turn the pages until I reach 'P'.

My body tenses with shock. Nestled amid the text of the doctors' notes is a small photograph of Maud.

Her eyes are pronounced, crescents of darkness beneath them. She looks tired. Her mouth is open, as if she's about to speak or ask a question, which makes me think she was confused, or not aware of what to do. I can see my own body in hers, tensed and searching for information to work out what is going on.

These photographs, placed at the beginning of each patient's record, were used for identification, but they're different from the mug shots or identity cards commonly used by institutions for the insane. Instead they are variations of the studio portrait, even if there is some strain evident in efforts to capture them. For example, Maud seems to be taking a breath. In another photo, a woman wears a straitjacket beneath her fur ruff.

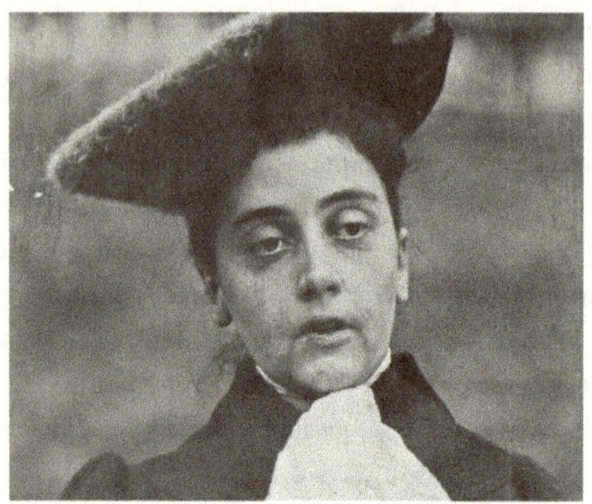

Maud at Holloway Sanatorium.
Surrey History Centre, 3473/3/6

The setting and structure of these photos, with patients dressed in their good clothes, suggests that the lives the patients had lost could be recovered, or at least emulated, within the sanatorium.[89] Rosa certainly thought Maud would get better, as she wrote to her American friend, the poet Louise Chandler Moulton, 'I fear she gets worse instead of better as I hoped she would do. One can only hope for the best, but it makes me very miserable.'[90]

The medical notes date from Maud's admission on 28 September 1902. They open with a description of her physical appearance: 'fairly developed but is slightly built – soft and flabby – Hair dark. Eyes brown.'[91] They state that she had been 'stone deaf since a severe attack of ScF [scarlet fever] in early infancy'. A few lines later, an account of her physical condition reads: 'She appears to be absolutely deaf – & speaks slowly & with some difficulty though she articulates correctly.' Her mental condition 'is difficult to ascertain on acct of her deafness – she lip reads to some extent & can easily read handwriting but does not speak readily'.

My hands start sweating in the white gloves. I had thought, given Maud's excellent literacy and ability to interact relatively well, that she might have had some hearing. Yet she had none at all. I take off the gloves and wipe my hands on my jeans. My mouth is dry.

Maud must have been exceptionally bright and hardworking to learn to read and write when she was completely deaf. She would have needed huge levels of concentration to learn words she couldn't hear, and she would have felt lonely and abandoned in the sanatorium because it would have been difficult for her to communicate and work out what was happening to her.

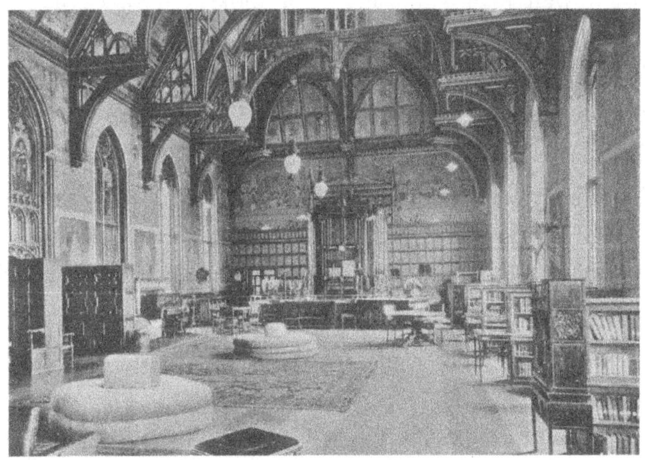

Recreation Hall, Holloway Sanatorium.
Surrey History Centre, 2620/6/26

I return to the notes. Maud informed the doctor who certified her admission that 'she is accused of killing her father & that the police are spreading reports of scandals about her – she cannot sleep & wishes to escape from the persecution'. Maud's behaviour is described as being 'difficult to manage – constantly trying to get out of the window with a view to posting letters – written to strangers'. She was clearly desperate to get away from the turmoil in her mind, either physically, by climbing from a building, or mentally, by trying to connect with people.

A few weeks after her admission, Maud seemed calmer. The notes state 'her deafness prevents her to a great extent from taking part in the community of the Hospital but she occupies herself with needlework & plays chess well'. Maud would have played this game in the Recreation Hall, a long, airy room with arching beams like a church's. Paintings of robed figures adorned the walls, and there were pianos and shelves of books. On top of the shelves a palm stretched from a pot. The windows let in a good amount of light, and electric lamps hung from the ceiling.

I imagine Maud with her chessboard, sitting next to a window or an electric lamp so that she had enough light by which to read her opponent's lips. She wouldn't have heard the echoes of feet or the rustling of skirts in that cathedral-like room, but she would have smelled sweat and body odours, or the scent of food drifting from the dining hall. Playing chess would have reminded her of her father who, she remained convinced, she was accused of killing.

In a letter to Rosa two months after Maud was moved into the asylum, Bulkley described a visit to his sister. Maud had been delighted by his gift of a packet of turquoise-headed gold pins, but she didn't ask about her mother or brothers. Her aunt Alice, Campbell's sister, had visited, and Bulkley asked, 'Were you pleased to see Aunt Alice?'

Maud ran her fingertips over the blue heads of the pins. 'No!'

'Why not?'

'Because she has been the cause of all the scandal!'

'There has been no scandal, Maud. Alice was very anxious about you, and made many enquiries, and had only come to find out how you were getting on.'

'Are you quite sure?'

'Quite, and you know she is very fond of you, and wants to do everything that she can for you.'

'Oh! I am sorry. Will you explain everything to her?'

'I will, but you should also write Alice a nice letter yourself.'

Maud pressed the end of a pin against her palm.

Bulkley tried again. 'How are you getting on here?'

'Oh! Very well, but sometimes they are rude to me and do not treat me like a lady. I was very angry with them, and stamped, and made a great noise, because they did not treat me properly.'

'It must have been a mistake on your part, Maud, and only your imagination. You must not pay attention to such things.'

'I was very angry with them, I told them I would not have such a thing, and I went like this at them.' Maud shook her fist, and laughed viciously.

Bulkley kept his voice even. 'I am sure no one meant to be rude to you, and I doubt it will happen again.'

Maud drifted to the subject of her father's death. 'It is absurd for people to make a fuss, for everyone knows exactly how he died. Bulkley, can you describe to me again exactly how it happened?'

As her brother spoke, Maud murmured in agreement. 'Of course it is all right, but I think a great deal about it; I cannot get over it.'

'You must not worry about such things, it's also over and past now, and it's merely your nerves being upset which makes you worry.'

'Yes, I think you are quite right, I must not think about it any more.'

As Bulkley left, Maud kissed his cheek. 'Thank you for the pins.'[92]

Although Maud seemed in good spirits on this occasion and said nothing about disliking the asylum, her doctor described her condition as 'variable'. In the gymnasium, where patients liked to go in the wet weather, Maud insistently took people by the arm and placed them in different parts of the building. She took Dr Moore's arm, too, and from this he surmised that Maud was trying to assert her authority.[93]

A year later, Maud had deteriorated. She often screamed loudly 'for hours at a time – she [had] marked delusions of electricity & attributes all sensations (such as tremor etc) to a "power thrown" at her by different people in her gallery'.[94]

My heart breaks when I think how Maud's deafness must have contributed to her paranoia. It would have been hard for her to communicate with people around her, particularly if they were strangers and didn't know how to face her and speak clearly so she could read their lips. Without reassurance, she wouldn't have been able to verify if her delusions were real or not, and she was certain that she was accused of killing her father, who had provided her with emotional stability and a familiar home. Thrust among people she didn't know, in a strange location, witnessing odd behaviour in the people around her, Maud would have been highly stressed. It is not surprising to read that six years later, in May 1908, she was 'confused with hallucinations of hearing and vague delusions of persecution' and was 'very difficult to understand'. At other times she was described as being quiet and coherent. 'Occupies herself well,' they wrote.

Meanwhile, Bulkley noted that to himself, their brother Geoffrey and Aunt Alice, Maud had 'either been suspicious or apathetic'.[95] Her doctor confirmed this, writing in his initial report that over the previous few months she had been 'indolent and apathetic with unreasonable prejudices against people, and has been rude to friends'.[96] The apathy suggests listlessness and depression.

I wonder about Bulkley's role in Rosa's decision to keep Maud in the asylum. Rosa was distressed about her daughter, but Bulkley counselled her, 'Nothing can be done, nothing altered. We have placed Maud in the best home that she can have. We know that she is getting the best care and treatment procurable. Beyond this we are powerless.'[97] A year later he wrote, 'I will always try to act for [Maud's] peace and happiness to keep her and support her in comfort, but I could never have her to live or stay with me.'[98] Perhaps, given the stigma of deafness and mental illness in the late nineteenth century, with its associations with animalism, Bulkley could not face caring for his sister.

Still, I can't help but think of Bulkley's comment in his letter complaining of Maud's behaviour at the D'Arcys' gathering a decade before: 'She'll have to make a break some time or other.' Nor can I get his dictatorial voice out of my head.

When Maud was placed in the sanatorium, Bulkley, then aged thirty, reiterated to his mother that she was not to visit, at least not initially, because to do so would 'probably confuse [Maud's] mind even more than it is at present' and would cause pain to both her and Maud.[99] In a letter of April 1905, Bulkley backtracked, responding to what must have been a plaintive note from Rosa. He wrote, 'If you are satisfied that it would be the best and kindest thing that Maud should pay you occasional visits, then I should feel deeply grieved if you did not have her.'[100] However, there is no record of Maud coming to stay with her mother. The tight threads that once bound them had been cut.

Humphrey's promise to take care of Maud never came to fruition. In a letter of January 1903 he referred to his mother's account of his sister as 'very sad'.[101] Some six months later he sent care of his mother a letter for Maud and a 'bead belt made by the Indians which I hope will please her. I bought it from the curio store in the big hotel where I am staying – they tell me all the American girls are wearing them, so it may be useful as well as ornamental.'[102] The next year, Humphrey died in a car accident in California when his passenger, a drunk, glamorous actress, took the wheel. Bulkley continued to manage the costs of Maud's care.

At moments of crisis, Rosa was precipitated into illness, and after Campbell's death she became unwell again. She burnt all of Campbell's correspondence. A prolific and inveterate communicator through letters, this act underscores just how distressed she was. It's not difficult to see how, given Rosa's state of mind, her strained relationship with Maud, her deference to Bulkley, and Maud's instability, the easiest solution for her was to admit Maud to an institution.

Over the ensuing years, Maud became increasingly incoherent. Her case notes from 1908 to 1926, held in a separate book, report her as experiencing 'auditory hallucination, at times noisy & violent'. Her doctors also reported that she suffered from constipation. Here was Maud, blocked up with all the things she couldn't say, her body screaming with the frustration of it.

Maud was transferred to the Sanatorium at St Ann's, Canford Cliffs, midway between Poole and Bournemouth, on 29 April 1912.

The management of Holloway Sanatorium believed in the therapeutic value of fresh air, so they purchased properties at Hove and Canford Cliffs for their patients.

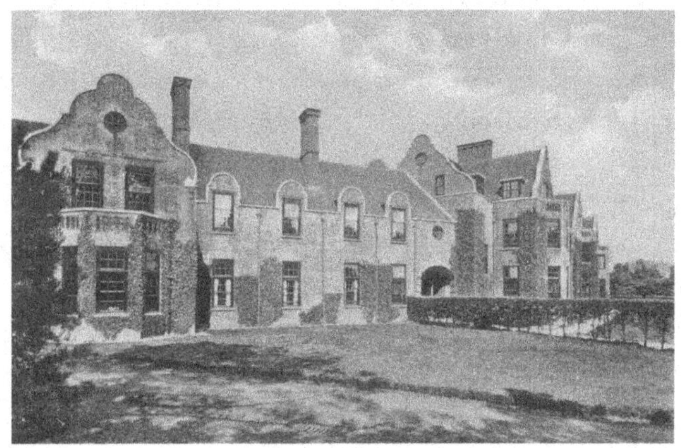

St Ann's, Canford Cliffs.
Surrey History Centre, 2620/6/26

Like Holloway Sanatorium, St Ann's is an elegant building of terracotta brick, although not as vastly proportioned. It is harmoniously laid out and attractive, with trees lining the grounds. The place would have been cold, particularly in winter. At the back of the building a track leads from the grounds down to the sea. As Maud liked nature, she likely walked along this track until she reached the shore. She wouldn't have heard the rush of waves or cries of gulls, but she would have felt the sea breeze on her face and smelled the salt. Perhaps in the summer she would have taken her shoes off and wandered in the shallows, ignoring the strange sounds in her head.

Most of the notes on Maud's condition from this period read, 'Still at Bournemouth.' On 20 June 1920 the notes record,

'She is deaf & dumb, mutters to herself and is an incoherent horror.' The final entry in Maud's case notes, dated 25 May 1926, states: 'Writes threatening letters that are incoherent but which bring[?] in the words "George & Mary" frequently. Is deaf & dumb but lip reads – makes loud noises like a peacock at times...The patient goes for drives.' I couldn't overlook the doctor's simile. As a person without speech, Maud was likened to an animal, slotting her into the long history of associations between deaf people and animals because speech was difficult for them.

Yet Maud still enjoyed being outdoors. Perhaps she looked at wrens fluttering in the hedgerows, or felt a soft spring breeze on her bare arms. Most poignantly of all, she was still trying to communicate through her mother's language as she had all her life, only now she was trying to write her way out of the asylum.

I shouldn't have been so surprised, then, to find a thick letter nestled among Maud's case notes. Written over twenty-two pages of stiff notepaper, it is dated 27 September 1905, three years after her admission, and is addressed to her doctor, Mr Moore. When I unfold the stiff paper, my skin prickles: here is Maud's adult voice, at last. As I begin to read, my stomach tightens.

The letter opens with Maud's plea for release: 'I have written to Mr Holden of Lackford Manor, asking him who should take me away from this Sanitorium [sic] as my Mother told me that she had nothing to do with me except the doctors, and my eldest brother.'[103] The lines brim with resentment. Maud appeals to a distant family member, Reverend John Shuttleworth Holden, the husband of her aunt Alice, rather than her mother. Later in the letter, she speaks of staying with Rosa, then unwell, until she was 'certainly better. I don't think she will want my company for some reason.' Whether this is an accurate representation of Maud's relations with her family is debatable, but Rosa's perceived distance clearly troubled Maud. Whatever their relationship at this point, what is clear is that Maud wants to go home. She begins with a request to leave, and her talk of departure takes up half the letter.

St. Ann's Heath
Virginia Water
September 27th 1905

Dear Dr. Moore,
I have written to
Mr. Holden of Lackford
Manor, asking him who
should take me away
from this Sanitorium, as

First page of Maud's letter to her doctor. Case Book, Surrey History Centre, 3473/3/6

There is a mix of orderliness and disarray in Maud's thoughts. After asking to go home, she writes:

> Perhaps it might interest you that my hearing is coming outright.

> Dr Mennell examined my left arm two months after my careless fire shock, and said 'Thanks to that except for another one.'
>
> I feel rather certain that it might come by itself, and that it could be done with skilful electric treatment. I ~~feel~~ am sure that it might give you and Dr Tinker a little encouragement, but I am unconxious [sic] of the new case.
>
> Dr Cumberbatch, the eminent oral surgeon informed Mother that ~~it might be~~ he had heard of such a rare case that he believed that I ought to read a great deal of history, and interesting things.

Maud's comments on her hearing suggest that she knew that to hear well – either immediately (outright) or correctly (out right) – was a prerequisite to being healthy. She was not impervious to the concept that to be deaf was to be deficient, or that she was at fault for being mentally unwell, as she writes towards the end of the letter, 'I believe that I cannot be looked down [on] by others for my very serious illness.'

Maud's thoughts veer from her hearing, to the 'careless fire shock', then back to her hearing, before slipping into books and reading. This lack of logical progression might indicate formal thought disorder, a type of psychosis. Maud's disordered thinking appears again when she writes, 'Please will you kindly ask Miss Carnaby to break off this lunatic electricity from the strangers as I don't desire my life to be known to them?' The mentions of lunacy and electricity might be a reference to electric shock therapy, which was used at Holloway.[104]

Maud's comments about her family are also revealing. Of Nancy she writes, 'I really realise that Mother strongly objects to my knowing Miss Harward's interests. I believe that she is doing good, but it seems so strange to think that she is really a misinformant as I expected her to say a single word about her progress – bulletin.' Nancy appears to be associated, on some level, with suspicion. By contrast, Maud refers fondly to Campbell: 'My deceased father always forbid any effort for me, and paid a great deal of invalid attention to my comfort, though he was very ill himself…I am so thankful to think that his last days were very happy indeed. It is unfortunate that he lost his wife's presence & I am sorry that he missed any confidence from his doctor. However he was on affectionate terms with her.'

In the midst of these comments, Rosa's status as a novelist flares brightly. Maud wrote drily, 'I am sorry to say I cannot agree with Mother's exciting novels, but perhaps you might have enjoyed one of them.' Instead, she would 'like to know something about insect and reptile life'. Maud's interest in the natural world, evident from her early letters to her grandmother about the excursion to the Natural History Museum, was still present.

Maud's final line reads, 'Will you allow me to join your company in presence of Mrs Holden one day? I am really satisfied with her correspondence.'

I carefully fold up the letter and close the heavy book of case notes. I return it with the gloves and walk out into the afternoon sunshine, heading along a canal. The light above my head is dappled by tall trees bowing over the path. Long reeds grow along the banks of the canal, boats moored beside them. I pass a woman walking a terrier and smile at her. I'm conscious of the soft light and air on my forearms, my sense of purpose in walking back to the pub at which I'm staying, the expanse of space around me.

For both Maud and me, writing was a way to stay in touch with people and gain pleasure from socialising when face-to-face interactions could be painful, bewildering and tiring. Other writers who have been deaf or hearing impaired have also been passionate and prolific letter writers, such as the Australian poet Judith Wright, who gradually lost her hearing from her mid-twenties. Mabel Bell, the wife of Alexander Graham Bell, wrote to her husband persistently, even though his replies were few.[105] In *The Woman at Home*, a monthly magazine edited by Annie Swan from 1893, female epistolary networks were recommended as a panacea for the loneliness of deafness.[106]

Rosa's career as a writer flourished as Maud grew up. Maud was eight when Rosa's third novel, *Nadine*, was published in 1882, making Rosa a sensation. The novel's protagonist has an illegitimate child and, when her lover dies of a heart attack, she drags his body down the hallway to avoid discovery. While wintering in Cannes, Rosa was invited to lunch with the prime minister, William Gladstone, and the Prince of Wales. The Prince told the prime minister's wife of *Nadine*, 'You must read Mrs Praed's book but you mustn't give it to your daughters.'[107]

Having seen her mother's success with writing, Maud might have imagined that it was a means by which one could access an interview with a prime minister and a prince, or release from an institution.

~

Not long after I find Maud's medical records and letter, Oliver announces he has a new job at a design firm in Farringdon in

London. I move out of the council housing flat at Broadway Market and join him in a terrace house in Stepney Green. The view from my desk is of our paved courtyard rimmed with a garden. Oliver comes home one Sunday laden with punnets of petunias from the nearby Columbia Road Flower Market. As I write, I watch him planting them, before he attacks the neighbour's vine that grows over our side of the fence. The neighbours are an elderly Italian couple; the husband is a florist who grows wattle in his backyard. In spring I watch it flower, wistful.

Living with Oliver again makes me feel more secure. My social life improves because I hang out with his friends, the way I used to in Sydney. Since we were children he has been a conduit to other people, repeating what they say and easing my anxiety about mishearing in conversations.

He also supports me financially, and I stop worrying so much about money. We gather a bunch of English and Australian friends into a book club named the Book Rangers (a pun on 'bushrangers'). I swim at the local pool at Limehouse, on the women-only evenings because it aggravates me when large men power past in the lanes, upsetting my tranquil laps. The blinds are drawn and the pool is full of Muslim women who hang on the ropes, chatting to one another.

Christmas comes around, and there is another White in London to celebrate. One of the cousins from the farm, who's travelling and working in the city, stays with us on Christmas Eve. The Italian neighbours play tinny Christmas tunes all through the night, keeping him awake. He steps into the bitter cold in his long johns and knocks on their door.

'I'm from next door. Could you turn your Christmas songs off, please? I can't sleep.'

They apologise. Silence falls upon the street.

The next day Oliver and I give each other the same Christmas present, a toy attachment for our phones that lights up when it rings.

'I think we're the same person,' I say. We laugh.

Our cousin helps us cook the roast, and after lunch we watch the Queen's message and *Doctor Who*.

I finally begin to breathe in London.

~

At UCL Library where I work, the loop system breaks down. It was installed when the issue desk was renovated, but was never loud enough and often crackled. I ask for a portable loop system instead, a sturdy plastic rectangle that will sit on the desk beside me. While I wait for it to arrive, my body works much harder than usual to hear.

'I'm exhausted,' I tell Oliver when I get home in the evening.

'When I was in Bristol, I went into a charity shop. The lady there wore a badge that said *I'm hard of hearing, please speak clearly*. You could try something like that.'

'I'll give it a go.'

The next day I ask the staff member in charge of printing if she can make me a badge. When it's ready, I pin it to my jumper.

The impact is negligible. Only a handful of people bother to modify the way they speak. One young man points to the badge and asks with a laugh, 'Is that a joke?'

I smile sweetly. 'No. I'm actually deaf.'

His own smile becomes uncertain, then disappears when he realises I'm serious. He drops his gaze, unable to look at me. Perhaps if I was elderly, like the lady in the charity shop, he wouldn't have laughed.

This incident doesn't bother me as much as the older, male academics who speak to me slowly and condescendingly. I complain to my boss at the time, leaning against the door of his office, 'Maybe I should get another badge and stick it on the other side of my chest. One that says, "I'm deaf, not stupid".'

'And then,' my boss replies, slapping his hand in the middle of his chest, 'you can have another badge here that says, "Stop staring at my tits!"'

I burst out laughing.

Although the technology I use tends to break and leave me stranded, I'm still grateful for the times it does work. Without it, I'd never have been able to study easily, travel, learn piano and flute, or talk to students in a library.

I became a cyborg soon after the visit to the audiologist in Sydney. Mum drove me to the National Acoustic Laboratories (now Australian Hearing Services) in Tamworth, a small, square brick building adjacent to the hospital. A receptionist's office adjoined the waiting room and there were another two rooms for clinicians. In one was a soundproofed glass room in which the hearing tests were carried out. I settled on a chair in this room and listened through headphones to a set of beeps ascending or descending in pitch or volume.

The audiologist marked down what I could hear on a graph known as an 'audiogram'. The graph for my right ear began with a line low on the left-hand side that ascended to a peak before dropping off dramatically, indicating that I could hear one small section of higher pitches quite well, although still not as well as someone with average hearing. The line on the graph for my left ear hovered near the bottom. It was decided, from looking at these graphs, that I should be fitted with a hearing aid in my right ear only. My left ear didn't have enough hearing to warrant an aid at all.

To make the mould, which was attached to the hearing aid by a thin tube, the audiologist piped cold, malleable plastic into my ear and bade me sit still. I watched him as he shaped the leftover plastic into a mouse, while he spoke to Mum. I couldn't hear their voices because my only working ear was plugged up. After a few minutes, he handed the mouse to me and gently pulled the mould, now firm, from my ear.

After the appointment, Mum and I visited Grace Bros, one of Tamworth's department stores. This two-storey building had the novelty of escalators and a cafeteria, where Mum bought hot chips and a chocolate milkshake for me, and a cup of tea and a sugared doughnut for herself. I slurped the milkshake, one hand sliding over the condensation forming on the tall tin cup, the other pushing the mouse across the table.

The mould for the hearing aid was sent away to be made, and it later arrived in a bulky envelope in the mail. Mum trimmed the tube, attached it to the hearing aid and squished it into my ear. I was now part-human, part-machine.

At my annual check-ups, I strained to hear the beeps in tests because, I reasoned with faulty logic, the more I could prove I could hear, the more normal I would be. Sometimes the sounds set off tinnitus in my head and I couldn't tell if what I was hearing was real or not.

In the waiting room, while we waited for the audiologist to analyse the results of the test, I gazed with longing at a poster of a woman's ear with a hearing aid in it. The hearing aid was studded with diamonds.

'Mum, can I have one of those?'

'No.'

'Why not?'

'They're too expensive.'

Disappointed, I kicked my heels against the legs of my chair.

At the time, the Australian government provided free hearing aids until the age of twenty-one. This benevolence was helpful when a hearing aid fell out of my pocket in the driveway and Mum drove over it. When I discovered it was missing, we went back to hunt for it. I found the aid in the dirt, flattened and cracked. I turned it on, dusted off the mould, and stuck it in my ear.

'Mum, it still works!'

She shook her head. 'You can't wear that. We'll have to go back to the hearing clinic.'

I was less lucky when, staying at Mum and Dad's in my early thirties, I left my hearing aid on the side of the couch's armrest while I made a cup of tea. When I returned, it was in hundreds of pieces. My parents' whippet gazed up at me blissfully.

'April!' I wrested the casing from her mouth in case it held the battery. The battery acid would have eaten through her stomach and I was pretty sure my father cared more about his dog than my hearing aid. I was no longer eligible for a free replacement and my parents generously found the cash for a new one. I kept it well away from the dog whenever I went home for a visit.

While my hearing aid helped enormously at school, I still had to concentrate hard to hear the teacher. The floorboards in the primary school at Boggabri were bare and every noise in the room, from chatter to scraping chairs, bounced off them. The school found funding to have the rooms carpeted, which made listening more bearable.

At age nine, my audiologist told my parents about a new piece of technology, a frequency-modulation transmitter and receiver system, or 'FM' for short. It looks like a miniature walkie-talkie set and involves the teacher wearing the transmitter – a small box that clips onto their belt or pocket, wired to a microphone on their lapel – while I pick up the sound through a receiver. When I turn my hearing aid to the 'T' (or telecoil) switch, it cuts out background noise and makes the speaker's voice intensely clear.

Mum took me to Tamworth again to try it out. I put the loop around my neck, switched my hearing aid to the telecoil setting and listened to the audiologist speaking into the receiver from the room next door. His voice was so clear it was magical.

Wearing the FM at school, I no longer had to lean forward to catch each word, or watch a face and lips with intensity to pick up their clues. I could listen to my teachers without lip-reading, which meant I could write without having to look up and watch them speak. My teachers' voices were wonderfully and compellingly lucid. Learning became a thousand times easier and more exciting.

In the mornings before school, I took the FM's batteries from their charger. In winter I liked their warmth and rolled them in my hand before slipping them into the transmitter and receiver. I gave Oliver the transmitter and he crouched with it on the other side of the table. 'Testing, testing.'

'Yep, it's working.' I bundled the pieces into their pouch and put it in my schoolbag.

My teachers usually forgot to switch the transmitter off when they went out of the room. Sometimes I'd listen to the principal speaking on the phone. If it sounded personal, I'd switch my receiver off, except for one occasion when he discussed the votes for school captain with the school secretary.

'Jess came in third.' He sounded surprised and I was stabbed by resentment. It dulled into the familiar, stale feeling of not being good enough compared to my brother, sister and four cousins, each of whom had been captain of the school.

At other times the FM was thrilling. In Home Economics in secondary school, my female teacher wore the transmitter when a male teacher knocked on the door. Seeing that we were occupied with writing in our exercise books, they retired to the kitchen beyond the classroom and I turned my receiver off. A few minutes later, they emerged. My teacher saw me, pointed and roared with laughter. I worked out that something had gone on in the kitchen, but I didn't know how to stop her laughing and explain that I hadn't heard it. Instead, I smiled.

Later, the teacher relayed the conversation to Mum. In the kitchen, she had been joking about a hole in her pantihose.

'Would you like me to sew it up for you?' the male teacher had asked.

When Mum repeated the conversation to me, we snickered.

Maud would probably have been too deaf for a hearing aid and FM system. Had she been born after 1982, she might have had a cochlear implant. This piece of technology is surgically implanted into the inner ear. It's connected to a transistor, which picks up sounds and converts them into signals that are sent through the skin to the implant, which in turn stimulates the nerves that send signals to the brain.

People often ask me if I'll get a cochlear implant. I've resisted because I've learned to cope with my residue of hearing. The thought of it also aggravates me. While technologies for FM systems, hearing aids and cochlear implants have revolutionised life for deaf people, at their heart lies conformity. Ads for hearing aids, which are becoming smaller and smaller, often use the word 'invisible'. Hearing loss is still something to hide, and a deaf person is still expected to act like a hearing person.

Parents of deaf children often prefer that their children learn their language of speech rather than sign. Andrew Solomon, in *Far From the Tree*, suggests it is difficult for parents to learn sign language because their brains are organised around verbal expression, and by the time they are of parenting age they have lost considerable neural plasticity. While this may be so, it doesn't mean that learning sign language is impossible, and the lifetime of effort a deaf child faces isn't much next to their parents' acquisition of a new language.

The argument around cochlear implants, Solomon continues, is part of a larger debate about 'the extent to which standardising human populations is a laudable mark of progress, and the extent to which it is a poorly whitewashed eugenics'.[108] Having become acquainted through Maud with the history of deaf education, and witnessed the degree to which this was influenced by social Darwinism and eugenics, it is difficult for me not to see cochlear implants as motivated by a desire to compel deaf people to communicate with hearing people on the latter's terms.

My audiologist tells me that there are cognitive benefits to be gained from cochlear implants, because they force the brain to keep processing sound and this wards off dementia, yet I still can't help but think that not much has changed since the nineteenth century: engineers are the new oralists, and they still force us to engage in the exhausting process of listening and speaking, which we can never do well enough by hearing people's standards. And hearing people rarely learn to speak the language of deaf people.

Before a lecture or a talk, I have to approach the speaker with my FM, tell them that I'm deaf, show them the equipment and explain how it works. I add that it doesn't record anything, because despite my explanations people still aren't sure what it is. Then I ask if they can wear it for me. Most are fine with my request, but others have been cautious or even suspicious, perhaps because I don't have a speech impediment, which to many is the marker of deafness.

The only time anyone refused to wear the FM was during my year on exchange at Berkeley. I enrolled in a course on women writers of colour and, before the first class began, I introduced myself to the lecturer, a small Asian woman. I explained, 'I'm deaf and this is an FM system which helps me to hear. Would you be okay with wearing it during the lecture?'

She looked at the small transmitter, frowning. 'I can't wear that! It changes the way I speak.'

'It only changes it for me, and I don't think I'll be able to hear you without it.'

She shook her head, but compromised by allowing me to leave it on her desk. I turned the volume on my hearing aid and my FM to their maximum. I could just hear her voice amid the now painfully loud rustling of pens and paper.

In retrospect, I wonder if I had not explained myself clearly, and if she had thought my FM would amplify her voice for the whole class, rather than just for me. Or perhaps she thought it was a tape recorder. Maybe my request had come across as an order, as I have a tendency to be abrupt. Either way, her response was puzzling, coming from an academic who espoused moving across borders.

When I related the incident to the support officer at the university's disability unit who was checking on me, he shook his head. 'By law, she has to wear it. I can speak to her if you like.'

I shrank at this. In the first class, the professor had explained with a smile that Asian people's surnames came first. I had smiled, too, enjoying her humour. I sensed there was some philosophical objection behind her decision, rather than obtuseness.

'I'll just put up with it.' A fellow Australian in the course shared her notes with me, as did another student who volunteered for the disabilities unit as a note-taker. When I checked my notes with theirs I found that I hadn't missed that much, but the energy needed to watch the lecturer's lips and face, combined with my anxiety about not hearing enough to get good marks, left me feeling like I'd run twenty kilometres without any training. Not for the first time, I wished that I could speak in sign language instead of having to carry out discussions in a way that brutalised me.

~

After her years of isolation in the asylum, Maud lost her skills of lip-reading. On 13 July 1924, after a visit to the asylum, Rosa wrote to her half-sister Dorothy that Maud, who was by this stage fifty years old, 'wants to say things and I can see she is losing her words. If she could be taught again, it would I am sure help her – the baffled, piteous look on her face when she wanted to say something and could not has troubled me much. Of course, she was constantly taught and kept up with things and now there is no one to help her lip-read or teach her.'[109] Even as early as

1913, Maud was having trouble being understood. An entry in her medical records states that she 'does not speak intelligibly for her ideas to be made out'. The loss of her words could be related to psychosis, as some sufferers have periods when they stop speaking or are unable to speak. Maud's medical notes also state that she had suffered from Graves' disease, an autoimmune condition that can have similar symptoms to psychosis.

In 1917, Rosa described to her stepmother Nora a letter from Maud's doctor at the sanatorium in which he stated that Maud needed to have her teeth out as they were 'in a condition injurious to her health'. Rosa could not bear the idea of this happening without Maud's consent but, she added, 'what is her consent!'[110]

Even prior to her admission to the sanatorium, and before her reason was damaged, Maud never had agency. She was a conscript to her mother's preference for oralism over sign language. Few recognised then – and arguably still do not recognise now – that deaf people have the right to choose how to voice themselves. For Rosa, a 'voice' was only something that could be heard. Instead of adopting sign language, a way of speaking that would have been easier for Maud, Rosa forced her daughter to learn her own, far more difficult means of expression.

Rosa toyed with the idea of teaching Maud lip-reading again in the asylum but decided against it for, she continued in her letter to Dorothy, 'It might also do her brain harm. I always feel that I may have over-exercised it by trying to teach her too much – She was very intelligent as a child.' Rosa could also see no point in it, adding that 'It would need infinite patience & to what end! She could never live in the world now.'[111]

I email Maud's letter and case notes to a psychologist friend, asking for her opinion. 'Maud's reaction to her father's death is profound,' she replies. A strong reaction to the loss of a parent is not uncommon, and an unexpected death has been associated with unravelling in vulnerable people, presenting as depression, anxiety, risk-taking or, in extreme cases, the development of delusions. In Maud's case, she was obsessed with the idea that she had been accused of killing her father and that she was wanted by the police.

If Maud had experienced paranoia, her thoughts becoming irrational and obsessive, my friend writes, 'it would have been hard for her mother to know what to do, and would have been unnerving'.

Usually, Rosa expressed subjects that preoccupied her through her fiction. Her novels are littered with incompatible couples trapped in marriage; domestic and racial violence; same-sex desire; and the overwhelming theme of spiritualism. Yet her distress over Maud only made its way into a few uneasy representations of disability. Her first novel, *An Australian Heroine*, ends with a description of the protagonist Esther's children – a son who is 'a fine, manly little fellow, and his father's companion out of doors'; and 'a lame girl, who is sensitive and dreamy-eyed, and resembles her mother in features'.[112] Her fifth novel, *Zéro* (1884), describes the heroine Varuna's torment in an unhappy marriage, and her gambling, which is motivated by her desire to find money to fund her deaf daughter's education. Echoing Praed's belief that Maud's deafness was a punishment for the wrongs of a previous life, Varuna exclaims to her love interest, George, 'I have sometimes wished, prayed, that my child might die. The maimed speech, the cramped intelligence, the dumb eyes, are living reproaches to me for a wrong unconsciously committed – reminders of an injury which I can never forget or forgive.'[113] By the novel's end, Varuna is granted her wish, and the child dies of an illness. Rosa's twentieth novel, *Madame Izàn* (1899), chronicles the romantic prospects of a young woman, blind since birth, who has recently recovered her sight. The woman's blindness is referred to repeatedly as a 'terrible affliction'.[114]

Given that, for Rosa, writing represented connection, her relative silence on Maud's deafness speaks of disavowal and regret, particularly when compared to her numerous fictional expressions of race, class and sexuality. Rosa's was a 'mute speech', to use scholar Jacques Rancière's idea that it is not just the lines of a text that speak, but rather a work's silent elements.[115] It seems that Rosa's pain on witnessing Maud's condition was so acute that it could not find expression in the usual modes of her novels. Rather, it could be heard only through a thunderous silence.

This is not to say that she was impervious to Maud's condition. In 1916 she and Nancy moved to Bournemouth so that it was easier for Rosa to visit, although this wasn't a permanent move at the time, as she and Nancy often travelled on the Continent for their health and a cheaper way of living.

Towards the end of Maud's life, it's difficult to tell how much she thought or felt, but a letter of Rosa's suggests she could remember previous acquaintances. In 1924, twenty-two years after Maud's admission to the asylum, Rosa brought a visitor, 'old Schnyder', to see Maud who, Rosa wrote, 'recognised her instantly, which astonishes me – after well over 20 years – was delighted to see her & we had quite a pleasant time sitting in those delightful grounds – S talking to her – then as usually happens she began to get excited & noisy & I had to take her in to the nurses. It is very pitiful.'[116]

In *The Art of Being Deaf*, Donna McDonald describes the physicality of being taught to speak. She and her classmates were instructed 'not through the dance of their hands, but through the effort of explosive vowels forced up through their sparrow-small chests and throats, and puffy, burring, hissing consonants shaped by their tongues and lips'.[117] Had Maud, when she was being taught to speak, become accustomed to being touched, and to touching others? In the asylum, did she yearn for her mother's affection and the comfort of her body? Did she remember the years of her teacher's hands pressing against her skin? Did she ever see deaf people signing, and feel longing in her fingers, the way her mother longed to hear the spirits from the afterlife?

~

In 1851, the year Rosa was born, the world's first undersea cable was laid between England and France, connecting the two countries. As her father moved the family around Queensland, buying and selling properties, telegraph wires were erected in each Australian state. Rosa grew up with telegraphs and, in a country as large as Australia, she was alert to the way they eclipsed distance.

In *The Romance of a Station* (1889), Rosa captured her experiences of living on Curtis Island nearly two decades before. Although this work wanders, as she explains, 'across the border-line into the misty cloud-regions of Fancy and Fiction…almost all the incidents are real, and even the most romantic of the episodes have their foundations in fact'.[118] On arriving at the island, Rosa's protagonist, Rachel Adsell, finds her romantic visions of the island shattered by a 'barren-looking and stony' shore and 'lanky unhealthy gum trees, with whiteybrown bark peeling off like scales, as if they were afflicted with some unhealthy disease'.[119] She encounters a storm of mosquitoes that 'offered a palpable resistance to one's hand, and their noise was as the roar of distant machines', foreshadowing a tormenting, hostile environment from which there was no escape.[120]

In real life, Campbell ran cattle on the island, but he was often away for business, leaving Rosa isolated and lonely. Clarke's research also indicates that Campbell continued a liaison with a woman with whom he was involved before his marriage.[121] By contrast, Rosa had a small baby girl, Maud, and little female company. In desperation, she turned to her dead mother for solace.

In Rosa's archive in the John Oxley Library is a piece of paper that begins with many crossed-out words, principally 'My' then 'no yes' following one another. The last uncrossed section before the letter starts is 'My yes yes'. It continues, with almost all of the words joined to one another, as follows:

> My dear Rosie
>
> Go to bed you are tired God loves you and will help you you were better this evening persevere and try to be bright and cheerful you had better go to Gladstone yes for a little time but do not stay too long your place is by your husband Stay till the McKennas go then you had better come back You are sleepy and I cannot write now Good night darling I am with you God is with you try not to be bad tempered tomorrow You will succeed in time and then you will be so happy only pray to God.[122]

This is a piece of automatic writing, purportedly created when a spirit enters a person's consciousness, takes hold of their pen and writes through their hand.

Clarke thought this response reflected Rosa's awareness, either conscious or subconscious, that there was no more possibility of escape from her marriage than there was of leaving Curtis Island, and that Rosa's helplessness may have influenced her own writing.[123] This points to the ambiguity of automatic writing, which exists, as Pamela Thurschwell writes in *Literature, Technology and Magical Thinking, 1880–1920*, 'on the cusp between inside and outside. Is it self-help? Is it a form of therapy? Is it like email? Is it more like talking to oneself or talking to another?'[124] Was Rosa actually hearing voices or was she writing to herself?

In *The Romance of a Station*, the only other female company on the island is Polly, the telegraph operator, to whom Rachel pays a visit. Polly is described as a 'shy, odd little woman of sixteen, reminding me somehow of a scrub kangaroo or a native bear, brought in and tamed, with her short, shaggy brown mane, her bright black eyes, her startled way'.[125] Despite never having left the island that formed her into this very local creature, Polly is a receptacle of global information. Through the telegraph, she acquires

> a mass of miscellaneous information, for the Cape was a through station, and all messages political, departmental, European, and otherwise, flashed along the line...Once, when the needle stopped for a minute, Polly announced in her abrupt manner: 'Mr Gladstone has announced to The House of Commons that in consequence of the vote on the

> Irish University Bill, Her Majesty's Ministers have tendered their resignations.[126]

Polly's *abrupt manner* and her habit of 'making long and short pauses on her words, as if she were keeping time to the telegraph needle', suggests that she is a Victorian cyborg, networked into what writer Tom Standage has described as 'the Victorian internet'.[127]

Yet for all her interest in unorthodox ways of communicating with the dead through reading and writing, it never occurred to Rosa that her daughter might more easily speak with her through the writing and reading of hands. Thomas Gallaudet, the co-founder of the first American school for the deaf, suggested that sign language could be perceived as a spiritual mode of communication. He admired the 'picture-like delineation, pantomimic spirit, variety, and grace…the transparent beaming forth of the soul…that merely oral language does not possess'. He also believed that sign language should be taught to the hearing in order to 'supply the deficiencies of our oral intercourse [and] perfect the communion of one soul with another'. It was a superior language to speech because of its expressiveness, and it brought 'kindred souls into a much more close and conscious communion than… speech can possibly do'.[128] Gallaudet's reference to communion highlights the intimacy of sign language, while his words *kindred souls* evoke the world of the spirits with which Rosa was enamoured, particularly after she met Nancy. It seems a terrible contradiction that Rosa could not see sign language's potential for communication, even as she was open to conversing with a spiritual world.

~

Our parents come to London for a visit. Oliver and I traipse with them across Waterloo Bridge to the Hayward Gallery to see Antony Gormley's *Blind Light* exhibition. Mum and I stand in the queue, looking at people coming in and out of the exhibit, a large glass cube filled with fog.

As soon as I step inside the cube, I panic. The fog is so thick I can't see anyone next to me. I rely upon my sight to orientate myself, and in the fog I'm blind.

'Mum, I can't see anything! I need to hold your hand.'

I find my mother's small, dry hand and she leads me to the glass wall. I slide my fingers over the cold surface, which is slippery with condensation, and follow the wall around until I find the exit. I step out, heaving in fresh air with relief.

I can't remember the last time I held my mother's hand. Neither she nor I are affectionate; she by nature, and me because I have taught myself to conceal my emotions, except in extreme situations and in my writing. But I'm glad for the fog, for my moment of panic. It meant I could hold Mum's hand once more, the way I'd clung on to her Indian cotton skirts or the loops of her large leather handbag when I was girl.

After our parents leave, my laptop blows up. In a tearful encounter at the Mac repair store near Spitalfields Market, I'm told it can't be fixed. I can't afford to buy another one. As the submission date for my research project is so close, Oliver generously lends me his. I type so much that I wear all the letters off his keyboard. He does my washing and cooks for me, and responds sympathetically when I complain how much I detest my work. My angelfish develops a growth and one morning I find her floating on the surface of the fish tank. Oliver scoops her out and buries her in the garden.

Watching him from my desk, I think of Hamish, who died and left a lacuna in our family. It was a blankness that was never discussed or addressed but that I somehow always sensed. Perhaps there was no point in talking of him; he was only eight months old when he died, a comet that flared across my parents' and sister's lives.

But then, in the galaxy of our family, another clump of hydrogen and helium appeared: a boy who loved Halley's comet, stuck glow-in-the-dark stars and planets on the ceiling, and Blu-tacked a chart of the planets to his wall. He orbited me, keeping me grounded with a gravitational wave. Or, to return to the Greeks, he was another *pharmakon*: we lost Hamish but gained Oliver.

Rosa and my mother endured much, and despite their ongoing grief they tried, like any mother, to do what they thought was best for us. Mum made a choice that was practical and that she thought would benefit me most: schooling at the local primary school with visiting support teachers, rather than teaching me sign language. Rosa, wanting Maud to socialise among hearing people, taught her to speak rather than sign. Had they known the emotional and physical cost of their choices, I have no doubt they would have thought differently. We were, however, daughters of strong-willed women who were determined that we would succeed, and this was the path they chose for us with the information available to them.

I try to keep this in mind when I think of Rosa these days, but even as I'm aware that she believed she was doing the best she could for Maud by placing her in a comfortable, salubrious institution, my relationship to her and her writing begins to change. Where once I had consumed her novels like lemon sorbet at the beach, now, when I re-read them, I see Maud sitting alone beside an asylum window in a shaft of sunlight, or waking screaming in a dark room, alert for the vibrations from the floorboards that meant a nurse was coming. Or standing by the window, a letter in her hand, waiting for her mother to take her home.

Maud died on 8 July 1941, surviving Rosa by six years. Her death certificate lists the causes as syncope (fainting), chronic myocarditis (an inflammation of the heart muscle) and artero sclerosis (now known as atherosclerosis, commonly referred to as a hardening of the arteries). She was sixty-seven years old and had been in the sanatorium for thirty-nine years. She outlived her entire family. The beneficiaries of her will were her cousins (the surviving children of Thomas de Montmorenci Murray-Prior); Elizabeth Jardine; and Alice Praed, the wife of Reverend John Shuttleworth Holden, the man to whom Maud had once written, asking to be released.[129]

Part of the tragedy of Maud's life was that she was simply born at the wrong time. In the 1970s and 1980s, the civil rights movement prompted a revolt against oralism. In 1987, the hearing president of Gallaudet University resigned. In the one hundred and twenty-four years since its inception, the university had never had a deaf president, and students made it clear that they wanted the next president to be deaf.

By mid-February 1988, the search committee narrowed the hunt to six candidates – three hearing, three deaf. On 1 March, three thousand people attended a rally at Gallaudet to indicate to the board of trustees that the Gallaudet community wanted a deaf president. Four nights later, on the night before the election, a candlelight vigil was held outside the board's quarters. On Sunday 6 March 1988, choosing between the three finalists, one hearing, two deaf, the board selected Elisabeth Ann Zinser, Vice-Chancellor for Academic Affairs at the University of North Carolina – the hearing candidate.[130]

The students were outraged. They demanded the resignation of the new hearing president and the chair of the board of trustees, and the reconstitution of the board with a fifty-one per cent majority of deaf members (it was at that time composed of seventeen hearing members and four deaf). They moved buses in front of the gates, which were barricaded with bicycle locks, and deflated their tyres. The lockout kept people from coming onto campus, while forcing the board of trustees to receive the protesters' demands. These were ignored, and the students walked on Capitol Hill. Seven days after the appointment of the hearing president, their demands were met. Elisabeth Zinser resigned and was replaced by I. King Jordan, Gallaudet's Dean of the College of Arts and Sciences, who was deaf. The deaf students had spoken loudly with their hands and actions, a visible presence to which the world listened.

The word 'belong' comes from the Old English term *gelang*, meaning 'at hand', or 'together with'. The Gallaudet students' use of speech with their hands indicated their belonging to a community of deaf people, and their desire to be led at by a person who was one of them.

It wasn't until 2010, at the 21st International Conference on Education of the Deaf in Vancouver, that a resolution was passed to formally reject the resolutions passed at the Milan conference, which stipulated that deaf children must be educated via speech, not sign.[131]

Around the same time the Deaf President Now campaign was underway, Colin Roderick, who wrote the first biography of Rosa, *In Mortal Bondage*, was preparing an inventory of the Murray-Prior Papers before passing them on to the National Library of Australia (he sold the material to the library in four lots between 1988 and 1991). It was a mammoth task, given the amount of material and the illegibility of many of Rosa's letters, and often he interpolated the inventory with his own comments. Against the record of Maud's first letter, he introduced her by writing, 'Alas! Maud lost her mind, became uncontrollable, had to be put into a mental asylum and became a vegetable.'[132] The first time I read this in the archives, I was aghast. This was the very mindset against which deaf people were campaigning as they fought for their autonomy, their rights and their voices.

The activism of the brave deaf people who campaigned for Deaf President Now paved a way for those who came after by reminding the hearing world that we are not animals or vegetables, that we do speak in a multiplicity of ways – writing, sign and speech – and that often, it is not deaf people who do not listen, but those who have all of their hearing. If society had listened to deaf people and learned their language, the way Abbé de l'Épée had learned from the two little deaf girls in the slums of Paris, so much heartache could have been avoided.

~

For a final hurrah before I leave London, Oliver and I dress in neon tights and skate beneath flashing lights at a roller disco in South London. I fall backwards and almost crack my tailbone on the floor. At Heathrow the next day, Oliver hands me a photo of us smiling at the camera in our rollerskates. I start sobbing, hug him goodbye, and don't stop crying until I'm halfway to Singapore.

My bruised tailbone is aching and I miss my brother already, but I'm going home at last.

3

Reading Hearts

On the twenty-four-hour flight back to Australia, the aeroplane stops to refuel at Changi Airport in Singapore. Instructed to disembark, we trudge out in silence, our eyes dry from hours of air conditioning and movies on tiny screens.

I've lost count of the airports around which I've walked in a jet-lagged daze, easing my aching calves. With my body on London time and the Asian clock reading eight hours ahead, it's difficult to work out where and when I am. At Changi there are purple Singapore orchids in white planters and soldiers with machine guns; at Suvarnabhumi the ceiling vaults in metal arches like a hangar's; at Kuala Lumpur the air conditioning is tepid. Otherwise the airports are the same: sterile, cavernous, consumerist spaces. Despite the plethora of digital clocks, there's little to show that time is passing; it's been wiped from the surfaces of glass, linoleum and chrome by silent workers. Often, for the few hours of wandering and waiting under bright lights, I don't feel real. I'm more like a ghost than a human being.

This experience is not new. As someone who belongs to neither the hearing world nor the world of deaf people, I'm constantly unsettled. Nor am I alone in this. Rhetorician Brenda Jo Brueggemann describes herself as being in a place between 'hard' and 'hearing':

> As one whose life has been spent always feeling one step behind in a conversation, usually caught in the exchange between two speakers and never quite 'there' at the moment any one person is speaking as I scrabble to process what I *have* heard, to fill in the many missing high frequency consonants that I *haven't* heard, to attend to ways that minimize background and interfering sounds, to construct a more accurate picture from the context surrounding the conversation (reading lips, attending to body language, noting facial expressions, trusting tone) – as such a one, I do anything but stand *still.*[1]

Like Brueggemann, I've always been 'one step behind' and never fully present in the act of hearing. Instead, I'm in a space between the present, in which words are being spoken, and the past, in which the words have been spoken but I must struggle to retrieve them by pairing them with context and body language. I am constantly journeying to find words and their context. I simply cannot *be*, nor am I quite *there*.

I wonder if this is the reason for my constant travelling. It's hard to settle when your body becomes accustomed to a state of constant vigilance, always seeking meaning and sensation, always reaching beyond itself.

I fly in to Brisbane with five hundred dollars to my name and a tooth that needs root canal therapy. I can't afford to live in Sydney, so my sister Bella offers me a room at her place. I make an appointment with a dentist and search for jobs.

The days are hot and bold, as though a designer has bumped up the colour. From Bella's verandah I watch storms roll in darkly and break upon the asphalt. I breathe in the smell of rain.

Bella is three years older than me. Hamish, the baby who died, lies between us. On the farm, I would sit at the table on the verandah, drawing or doing my homework. Whenever Bella walked past, she would poke me, pull my plaits or flick her finger behind my ear.

'Bella! That's not fair. I couldn't hear you coming up behind me.'

She would laugh and run away.

As adults we've mellowed, and I've learned to control my irritation. Besides, she now has kids of her own to aggravate instead. They are animated, active little creatures. My nephew waits for me to get out of bed each morning. When I open my door and stagger out, he dashes to his mother, shouting, 'Mummy! Auntie Jess is *awake*!'

As I put my breakfast together, blinking sleep from my eyes, he stands next to me and prattles. I make appropriate noises in what I hope are the right places, unable to hear what he's saying because I don't have my hearing aid in and it's far too early to talk.

In the school holidays, Bella and I take the children to see *Happy Feet* at the South Bank cinemas. I queue for tickets, then explain to the sales attendant, 'I'm deaf. Does the cinema have a loop system or some other kind of technology to help me hear the film?'

'I'll just check with the manager.'

The girl returns. 'I'm sorry, we don't have a loop system or headphones.'

I frown. 'Don't you realise that, by law, they need to be installed?'

The girl looks abashed. 'This is an old cinema. It will cost us too much to put one in.'

I take the tickets and relay the conversation to Bella.

'What!' she explodes. 'Christ, they're useless.'

I shrug. The girl's response is common. I'm inclined not to bother with complaining because it takes energy, but once an audiologist in London told me, 'If you complain, you make it easier for the next deaf person who comes after you.'

Eight years later, as I finish writing this book, I go to the same cinema again to watch *La La Land*.

'I'm deaf,' I tell the sales assistant. 'Do you have a loop system in the cinema?'

'No, I'm sorry, we don't.'

It's too much; I turn around and walk out.

Back in those overheated days following my return from London, I borrow some money from Bella for the dentist. He fixes the stabbing in my jaw and I start running again. There's a creek that meanders near her house, mangroves and gums growing thickly over it. In the mornings fruit bats roost in them, screaming as they settle into sleep. At the end of the day, they awaken and unfurl against the sky like a black flag, squealing as they rise. It takes me a while to work out that it's the bats making the noise. I keep checking over my shoulder for a child squalling in a stroller.

Each afternoon, Bella comes home from work and regales me with stories of her day, acting them out with panache and expression. She's a loud, vivacious woman, and sometimes people don't like that.

Before I left for London, she stayed with me in Sydney for a weekend. On a hunt for her wedding shoes, we caught a bus to Bondi Junction. Out of habit, Bella raised her voice to speak to me. Partway through the conversation I realised she was no longer talking to me, but to a thin woman sitting behind the driver who had turned to her and shouted, 'Do you have to speak so loudly that the rest of the bus can hear?'

'Yes, I do! My sister's deaf.'

The bus pulled over by the side of the road at a stop.

'I've paid for my ticket,' the woman continued. 'There's no reason why I should have to listen to you. You can get off there.' She pointed to the bus's open doors, beyond which was a bus shelter.

'I just *explained* to you, my sister's deaf. I've paid for my ticket too. Why don't *you* get off?'

The woman bunched up her mouth and turned her back. Cautiously, the bus driver pulled away from the kerb. I was amazed and impressed by my sister; I could never come up with ripostes that fast.

I also figured it wasn't the time to tell her she was so loud I could hear her without my hearing aid.

Following a handful of job applications, I'm invited to an interview for a research assistant position at a not-for-profit organisation that supports people with autism. Although I know little about the condition, I figure my research skills might be useful.

In an airy room facing a garden, I sit opposite the human resources manager and the head of research. The latter is a softly spoken woman and I have to lean forward, straining, to catch her question, 'Why is it important that we focus on the communication skills and education of children with autism?'

I think of my own days at school, when I sat on the bench by myself beneath the jacaranda, reading. 'So that they feel less alone.'

A few weeks later, I begin the new job and pay my sister back for my dental work.

Along with some financial stability and the high, clear days, there are other pleasures. I join the local library and cycle to the pool at Stones Corner. I drink good coffee at outdoor cafés, a book open before me. My skin darkens and my calves harden. I remember what it's like to be happy.

I have opted for part-time work so that I can keep writing. Not long after I'd begun *A Curious Intimacy*, I had the idea for my second book, which will become *Entitlement*. It has been sitting in my head for six years.

After living in Surry Hills in the early 2000s, I moved into a terrace in Paddington with a historian. Once she asked me, 'Do you realise that your life of privilege has come from land that belongs to Aboriginal people?'

I chewed my lip. 'I haven't thought about that before.'

I began to pay more attention to politics. I read the *Bringing Them Home* report about the Stolen Generations, Aboriginal and Torres Strait Islander children who were removed from their families and placed with white families or in settlements. I was aghast that I'd not known any of it. At primary school, all we'd been taught about Aboriginal Australians was how they made bark shelters and what tools and weapons they used.

I read about native title, the recognition by Australian law that Aboriginal people have rights to their land. The foundational case was *Mabo v Queensland* in 1992. One year after this, the Australian Prime Minister, Paul Keating, formalised the recognition of the concept of native title through the Native Title Act.

Bella had moved to Brisbane after she met and married a man of the Yugambeh people.

I ask her, 'Could there have been a claim for the farm?'

'I overheard Dad and his brothers talking about that when Mabo passed. But no, they couldn't, because you need to have proof of unbroken descent.'

'What do you mean?'

'Aboriginal people need to show proof that they've stayed on their country since British colonisation and that their connection to that country is unbroken.'

'But that's impossible! They were forced to move.'

'I know.'

I bristle.

In the room in my sister's house, her cocker spaniel Bentley sitting on my feet, I begin to write about a brother who is missing, for Oliver is still back in England. I draw on my visceral sense of homesickness in London; of my understanding and experience of colonisation; of not having my own language and of the ambivalence and power of using and enjoying a dominant culture's words; of being tightly woven into a history of assimilation that made it hard for me to recognise myself as deaf. I try to write about reparation to Aboriginal Australians, about making up for a terrible loss, about coming home.

As I write, I'm troubled. Like Rosa, my forebears were pastoralists, and I have little doubt that their actions were similar to her father's. When Rosa was six and living at Naraigin (also known as Hawkwood) station, eleven Europeans on the nearby Hornet Bank station were killed by Yimin people, probably in retaliation for the abduction of Yimin women. In reaction, the settlers, led by Rosa's father, Thomas Murray-Prior, massacred the Yimin. The number of Aboriginal casualties was estimated to be more than five hundred.

A few pages into her autobiography *My Australian Girlhood* (1902), Rosa states baldly,

> I love the Blacks. Some of them were my playfellows when I was a child at Naraigin, up in the then unsettled north; and truly, I think that the natives have not deserved their fate nor the evil that has been spoken of them. It was mainly the fault of the Whites that they learned treachery, and were incited to rapine and murder.[2]

In her novel *Fugitive Anne*, published the same year, Rosa expressed her ambivalence about colonial violence. Her protagonist Anne is unable to reconcile her sympathies for the Aboriginal Australians who have suffered brutalities with those for the white colonisers. Anne finds 'Her brain was dazed, her senses numbed, the future was a blank.'[3] The novel then leaps into the fantastic, a genre that combines the marvellous and the real. Rosa describes Anne and her Aboriginal companion Kombo travelling into the centre of Australia, where they discover a lost race. Through this imaginative trajectory, Rosa creates a fictional lineage for white settlers without having to confront the annihilation of Aboriginal people and their culture, and her family's role in this.[4] It wasn't the only occasion on which Rosa used this genre to write about an issue that was difficult for her to resolve. She also used the fantastic to express her love for Nancy by relocating it to the world of ancient Rome.

I live in the twenty-first century. I have some sense of what colonisation feels like through being assimilated into a mainstream culture, although at the same time I have been privileged by the stolen land on which I grew up, as well as my access to technology and my family's tireless efforts to support me. Evading reality is not an option in this book.

~

My boss, who has worked in the disability sector for forty years, tells me about a former colleague who has been deaf since birth and has incredible lip-reading skills. 'I had lunch with Donna and some friends. A person was speaking and their head was half-turned away, but Donna could still work out what they were saying!'

I send Donna an email. On a bright day in July 2010, a year or so after I've returned to Australia, I make my way across the campus at the University of Queensland at St Lucia to meet her.

A friendly looking woman with short, peppery hair is sitting at a table beneath the patchy shade of palms. I approach her. 'Donna?'

Her face brightens and I pull out an unsteady chrome chair. When our coffees arrive, I listen intently as Donna describes the memoir she's writing for her PhD, which explores the impact of deafness and of being deaf on her life. She attended the Oral Deaf Pre-School in Yeronga, then the Gladstone Road School for the Deaf in Dutton Park. When she was eight, she was enrolled in a mainstream school with hearing students. Her memoir is framed by her reconnection with her friends from the Deaf School.

'It's unusual,' Donna continues, 'that you're good with words. Many deaf people aren't.'

'Really?' I think of the long journeys in the car between school and music lessons and the audiologist, the way books assuaged my boredom and loneliness, how writing had helped me to express myself and connect with people. To me it was logical that one should turn to reading and writing when listening was so hard.

When I thought about it more, Donna's comments made sense. For those who sign, writing is foreign because sign language has no written counterpart. Spoken English also has tricks tucked into it, such as the silent 'p' in 'psalm', that don't correlate with what is on the page. Some deaf people are understandably resistant to a language that, as scholar Jennifer Esmail points out, 'carries its own pejorative resonances for terms such as *deaf*, *dumb* and *mute*'.[5] Esmail also notes that deaf people of the nineteenth century 'were typically signers first and writers second, yet they were forced to use written English to represent themselves textually'.[6]

English was Maud's first and only language. She would have undertaken hours of difficult practice to transfer the shape of a person's lips to the page, to objects around her, and back to her writing. If I, who had some hearing, found it tiring to lip-read, then Maud must have been utterly exhausted.

Even at Gallaudet University a century later, students were expected to become skilled in both American Sign Language (ASL) and standard written English, even though, as rhetorician

Brenda Jo Brueggemann writes, 'ASL and English differ radically – syntactically, conceptually, modally – in almost every way' and ASL has no written component.[7] Again, I see links with how Aboriginal people have been treated. Their language, too, was taken from them, and they were punished for using it. Deaf children at school would have their hands slapped if they were caught signing.

Beneath the palms, Donna and I move on to our mutual hatred of hairdressers who try to talk to us despite hair dryers roaring in the background.

'I tell them what I want done, then I say, "No, I don't have a boyfriend," and then I read my magazine,' Donna says.

I laugh with delight. Never have I felt so comfortable with someone within a few minutes of meeting them. Here is a woman who understands what it's like to strain to hear, to be mocked for something you've heard incorrectly, who knows you have to say no to events to conserve energy, no matter how much you want to go out, because trying to hear will be too draining.

Donna is also a writer. In 1991 she published *Jack's Story* about the loss of her son from SIDS and her management of the intolerable grief that followed. She is also recovering from chemotherapy for a bout of cancer. She's an incredibly strong woman.

We get onto the topic of romantic fulfilment.

'I've had terrible luck with men,' I admit. 'I'm too self-sufficient.'

'You're a lot more confident than I am when I was your age.'

'Am I?'

'Yes. But the self-sufficiency, that's my problem, too. You have to be, when you're deaf. You have to be independent and to learn to look after yourself, and not all men find that appealing.'

Once again I have the sense of something settling into place, like a bird alighting in a tree, its wings relaxing. When I say goodbye and walk back past the sandstone buildings to the bus stop by the lakes, my step is buoyant.

How is it that I've reached the age of thirty-two and this is the first, extended conversation I've had with another deaf person?

I didn't properly realise that I was deaf until I was twenty-one, on exchange at Berkeley. During that year away I felt my sense of self shifting and opening, like petals arching in the sun. I spoke to people because I often needed directions and, after each interaction, my confidence surged. I found a job that I enjoyed in the Bancroft Library in the middle of the campus, and worked among gentle people who liked books. Making money to cover my living expenses made me feel competent. As I was discovering new places and elements of myself, I decided to see a psychologist. On some subconscious level, I knew my psyche needed exploring as well.

The psychologist had a broad, open face, and her round body and folded hands radiated calm. In the first session, she asked. 'What brings you here, Jessica?'

'My parents are paying for health insurance while I'm here so I figured I should use it.'

She contemplated this. 'Usually people have a specific problem they want to solve.'

'Do they?'

'Yes.' She smiled.

'I'm deaf, and I think that's caused some problems.' Hesitantly, I explained my anorexia and constant apprehension about failing to perform well. As I spoke, she scrawled in her notepad.

In the middle of the year I had moved into a large share house called a co-op. It was run in part by students who lived there, who did housework and cooking to keep the costs down. I shared a room with two girls, both from San Diego. One invited me to her family's place for Thanksgiving.

Although I was charmed by San Diego's blue skies and sharp winter air, I was worried about being a burden, and that I was not entertaining enough for my friend. I wondered if she had only invited me so that I wouldn't feel alone.

'On Thanksgiving Day,' I said to the psychologist, 'all my friend's relatives were there. I didn't know what to say to anyone, and I couldn't overhear any conversations so I couldn't join in. I felt like a failure —'

'Jessica!' She brought me up short. 'You're deaf.'

In the dimly lit room, I looked at the kind, generous woman opposite me, her cheek glowing from a lamp on a small table to her right. Within seconds, I realised that a huge amount of my daily anxiety came from my expectation that I act as a hearing person. Constantly checking body language, listening for cues in conversations so I knew when to respond, straining to hear and lip-reading, were all mechanisms that I relied upon heavily to pass as a hearing person, instead of simply explaining that I was deaf and asking people to speak more clearly. No wonder I was always so tired; the constant vigilance was exhausting. Not only that, but I blamed myself for failing to interact with others as smoothly as someone with all their hearing.

The day after this conversation, I sat in my favourite coffee shop, Caffè Strada, a pile of notes for an essay beside me. I couldn't concentrate on the essay. I was trying to figure out where my unreasonable expectations of myself had come from. Part of it, I realised, was my family. As I'd grown up, I'd had no role models other than the bunch of show-offs who surrounded me.

When our parents, aunts and uncles partied in town or on other properties, we kids were left with our grandparents. Sometimes it was all nine of us, sitting out the front of the house in the evening playing charades. Our grandfather's dogs panted in the spiky grass and crickets whirred. I detested charades because I couldn't hear the suggestions that my siblings or cousins yelled out, so I never won. Usually I fell silent, the cement step hard and cold beneath my bottom.

In winter we headed indoors and raided the dress-ups box, which stretched the length of my grandmother's sewing room. Draped in satin gowns and moulting stoles, the girls glided into the living room, their chins held high. The boys, in tweed jackets and caps, hobbled behind on walking sticks. I pulled on a pale green dress of my grandmother's, the long sleeves hanging over my hands, and followed my cousins into the living room. My grandfather's blue eyes lit up at the sight of us all.

His sons were born performers. At university, the youngest played in a band named The Rubber Extenders. My father was always singing Gilbert and Sullivan songs around the house, and played Judas in a Gunnedah production of *Jesus Christ Superstar*, jigging a rockstar dance in white cotton pyjamas. Meanwhile, their elder brother donned a red jacket and breeches to become Gunnedah's Town Crier. It was little wonder, then, that their kids were always talking, singing, playing an instrument, or all three. It was expected that I would be a performer as well, regardless of having lost most of my hearing.

All the White children learned an instrument when they were young. I took piano lessons with Mrs Rose, who lived on a property outside Boggabri. As she lived closer to town than us, she picked my cousin Naomi and me up from the bus after school.

At her kitchen table, she gave us a slice of orange cake and a glass of milk.

'Is there any chocolate cake?' I once asked.

'No. Don't you like the orange cake?'

I looked down at the table. It was bad manners to complain that I was tired of orange cake. 'No, it's fine.'

While Naomi had her lesson, I splashed in the pool, climbed up to the widow's walk at the top of the house, or wandered through the stand of she-oaks at the back of the garden, their fallen fronds making a spongy carpet beneath my feet.

I was good at piano because I did my practice, but I had little flair. I could hear the treble better than the bass, as the pitch was higher and the residue of my hearing that remained was in my right ear. I liked learning the Italian words on the score, delighted Mrs Rose with one hundred per cent in my first musicianship theory exam, and won competitions at the Gunnedah eisteddfod. I was told, however, that I didn't have enough hearing to match my voice to a tune. Instead of singing a melody in my exams, I was given extra sight reading (reading a piece of music and playing it straight away).

When I was older, I grew resentful of not being allowed to sing, just as I resented my mother's decision that I shouldn't learn languages because they were too hard. Why should *hard* factor into anything, I thought, when my entire life was a strain? At the time, however, I was too young to think for myself and I did what Mum said.

I practised doggedly on the antique Blüthner piano in my parents' bedroom, pausing in my scales to stare into space and daydream, or muse over the paintings on the wall around me: a naked woman, her back to the viewer, with a wash basin, and my great uncle's oil painting of Mount Aspiring in New Zealand.

Outside, next to the verandah, was the tankstand. It supported a rainwater tank and a yellow banksia rose that Mum planted beside it. Sparrows liked to sit in its thick foliage, and their high-pitched twittering drove me mad. Sometimes I charged outside and threw stones at them to give myself some peace as I played. They would start up again a few minutes later.

Mrs Rose put together a production of *Toad of Toad Hall* in Boggabri when I was twelve. The nine White children were in the cast. One cousin was Badger, another Toad. I was invited to be a rat. I fidgeted through the rehearsals. It was dusty in the old Art Deco hall, and a heat rash bubbled in the crook of my arm. For me, acting mostly involved standing around. I couldn't hear what was going on.

'I don't like it there, Mum. It's boring,' I complained.

'You don't have to stay if you don't want to, but you'll need to tell Mrs Rose yourself.'

After the next rehearsal, before we filed out of the hall into the cooling afternoon, I approached my music teacher. 'Mrs Rose, I don't want to be in the play any more.'

She frowned. 'If you leave, Jessica, I'll be very disappointed.'

I weighed up my boredom against her unhappiness. 'I don't want to do it.'

There were also end-of-year school plays to endure. In Year Five I was an angel, dressed in a shift made from white cotton trimmed with tinsel. At the dress rehearsal, I stood up without thinking and spoke my lines. A few minutes later, I did the same again.

That evening at bedtime Mum asked, 'Did you realise that you said someone else's lines today?'

'What?'

'Your teacher said you got up twice.'

'Oh!' I recalled the ripple of discomfort I sensed among the students as I sat down after saying my lines. 'I must have said Paula's as well.'

My mother laughed and switched out the light. I lay awake in the darkness, wondering what had happened. I'd been so bored during the play that I'd memorised all the lines until I thought they were my own.

Thinking about this in later years, I'm not surprised. I wasn't simply bored; I was also a born performer like the rest of my family. I just didn't know it then.

Although I could never match the wit and verve of my cousins, I still wanted to prove that I could speak and act as well as they could. Inspired by some of them who were taking elocution lessons, I pestered Mum to enrol me in the speech section at the Eisteddfod.

Under the bright lights of the stage, which made the audience difficult to see, I proudly recited a poem about a lamb. To my amazement, I came second. I strained to listen to the adjudicator.

'You would have come first,' he said, 'except that you forgot the entire second stanza.'

My smile was huge. I didn't care that I had forgotten the stanza. I'd proven that I could speak well enough to pass as a person with all their hearing. I was camouflaged as a 'normal' person.

This meaning of the word 'normal' entered the English language around 1840.[8] It had previously meant 'perpendicular', which suggests correctness and uprightness, but the emerging field of statistics shifted its associations to those of conforming to a standard.

Belgian statistician Adolphe Quetelet (1796–1874), a teacher of mathematics and a student of astronomy, observed how astronomers located stars using a 'law of error'. They plotted all the sightings of a star and averaged the discrepancies. This gave him the idea of an 'average man', which was the average of all human attributes in a given community.[9] Having deemed that there was an average man, it followed that there was an average society made up of average inhabitants. Disabled bodies, which are not average, began to be excluded.

In the unstable world of 1830s revolutionary Belgium, Quetelet longed for a sense of control, and this shaped his belief that a single method of enquiry could be applied to the natural world, to society or to criminal behaviours. Across the channel, meanwhile, another flurry of interest appeared. Monitoring people through the Reform Act (1832), Factory Act (1833) and Poor Law (1834) resulted in the formation of the Statistical Society of London and the Royal London Statistical Society.[10]

Quetelet arrived at this notion of the 'norm' through astronomy, a field based upon sight. He transferred a process used to map suns at an immense distance onto humans. It is therefore not unexpected to find Lennard Davis, a scholar whose parents are deaf, observing that almost all the early statisticians were eugenicists, as eugenics was also driven by the sense of sight. 'Disability,' Davis writes, 'is a specular moment.'[11] Those who do not look like the dominant culture are viewed with suspicion or disgust, whereas those who 'pass' as 'normal', such as deaf or dyslexic people, can do so because of their appearance.

Somehow I knew this when I was a teenager, driving myself to lose my puppy fat because I thought it would make me desirable. If I was desirable, I would find a boyfriend. If I had a boyfriend, I would be accepted. This spurious reasoning never worked, as I never found a boyfriend. When we moved off the farm, I steadily put back on the weight I'd lost, so that I became as plump as I had been a few years before. Developing an eating disorder didn't resolve my underlying issues of persistent anxiety, lack of confidence and an inability to communicate well. A few years later, though, I realised that my appearance could work in a different way: as armour.

'The ugly duckling has turned into a swan,' my uncle said when we visited the farm the Christmas after I began university. This uncle had three boys, and as a child I sometimes stayed with them while my parents were away. My aunt brushed and braided my hair before school while my uncle stood by with his cup of tea, watching. Once, he reached out and touched my hair.

'It's so soft,' he marvelled. I realised he didn't know what it was like to have a daughter with long hair.

My uncle's expectations that women should be beautiful echoed my father's. They weren't uncommon in our conservative rural community. In later years, seeing the damage that had been done, Dad tried to be more circumspect in his comments.

That Christmas, I was nearly nineteen. It was the year I started university and stopped eating. As my weight slid off, I found I had a figure. In the mirror attached to the door of my cupboard, I looked at my bust and narrow waist, speculating. For the first time in my life, I had noticed men looking at me. Having believed for all of my life that I was unattractive, this revelation made me stupidly proud.

My endless peregrinations diverted into clothing boutiques in town. I had an allowance from my mother that didn't extend to clothes, but I still tried them on. I found a new delight in touching silk, lace and elastane, and seeing which colours suited my skin. Soon, a passion erupted for the delicacy of stilettos, patterned handbags, the scroll of flowers and leaves on a skirt. It was also more than this: a performance of normality that, I thought, kept me safe.

Over the years, I have acted this role of a hearing person too well, to the point where people don't realise that I'm deaf unless I tell them. One evening a few summers ago, at my local bookstore Avid Reader, I waited for a book launch to begin. A man approached and gestured to the empty seat beside me. 'Do you mind if I sit here?'

'Not at all.'

In his hand was a copy of Graeme Simsion's *The Rosie Project*.

'I enjoyed that,' I said. 'I thought it was funny.'

'I don't think it's right to make fun of people who have a disability.'

'That's true. But if you have a disability, you need to be able to laugh at yourself. I'm deaf, by the way.'

'Really? Do you have an implant?'

'No!' I remembered Donna McDonald's annoyance when someone told her, 'You don't look deaf.'

I don't have an obvious speech impediment. In the years after I had meningitis, my voice was flat. My family worked relentlessly on correcting my pronunciation, and my visiting teacher for the deaf, Mrs Matthews, taught me how to put intonation into my sentences. In my twenties, before I'd even gone to England, people asked me, 'Are you English?'

'No,' I would tell them. 'I'm deaf and my family worked really hard on my speech.'

I have often wondered if something else was going on. Was it my father's wistful musings on the greenness of England? Did a colonial hangover make its way into my voice?

'Don't speak like that; it's common,' my father reprimanded me.

'Don't use "but" at the end of a sentence; it's common,' said my grandmother.

'You're starting to sound common,' said my mother when I started high school. I'd developed a twang that I couldn't hear.

Or was it much more straightforward: that my parents, like Rosa, wanted me to have the best possible start in life, and this was how they thought it could be achieved? As extroverts, they knew no other way to be.

Ever eager to please, I did what they told me and monitored my voice as best I could.

After the exchange with the fellow in the bookstore in Brisbane, I made a decision to stop explaining to people that I was hearing impaired, as I usually did, because the word 'impaired' suggests deficiency. Instead, I explain, 'I'm deaf. I have no hearing in my left ear and half in my right.' This, I hope, conveys the extent of my hearing loss, while expanding people's understanding of what deafness is, for it isn't always a person who signs. Deafness is a range of hearing losses in different registers, and each deaf person has a unique way of interpreting and representing their world.

There are two models of deafness: a cultural model and a medical model. 'Deaf', as a proper noun, was first used by James Woodward in a paper in 1975, in which he stated, 'Throughout this paper, the convention of capitalising the word "Deaf" is utilised when the word refers to any aspect of the Deaf community and its members. Uncapitalised "deaf" refers to the audiological condition of deafness.'[12] Deaf people do not see themselves as having a disability. Rather, deafness is a culture with its own language and history, much like that of Italians or of New Zealanders.

Woodward's use of deaf/Deaf was never meant to be a taxonomy, for people can be both deaf and Deaf at the same time. At times the distinction has morphed into an either/or situation, which can be divisive. While I understand the solidarity and comfort that comes from being part of a community, particularly for members of the Deaf community who have been scolded and scorned for not speaking well, and while I feel an affinity with Deaf culture and am grateful for the activism, efforts and consciousness-raising Deaf people have achieved, I am also wary of that slash, its potential for division.

Rather than identifying as Deaf (at least at this point in time), I consider myself as having a disability. I don't see this as a negative thing, although most of our society does. Rather, I see my disability as something that has given me a unique outlook on the world, and made me more empathetic. While I have suffered on account of it, this is not because of my hearing loss but because of the attitudes of the people among whom I move.

These realisations have been part of my 'coming out' as a deaf woman, a phrase I encountered in rhetorician Brenda Jo Brueggemann's book *Lend Me Your Ear*. Like me, Brueggemann believed she should act as though she could hear. Then she started taking sign language classes and went to Gallaudet University and, at the age of thirty, 'came out' about her deafness, akin to a gay or lesbian person coming out. She describes the similarities between deaf and queer culture:

> Deaf people have often been curiosities, 'queer' in their 'strange' and 'silent' way; gay people have

> just as often been silenced, speechless in dominant heterosexual histories and discourse. From these positions, deaf and gay individuals 'pass' – playing out and through a politics of passing, balancing borders of (non) existence in their daily interactions and relationships...Hearing, like one's sexual orientation and relationships, cannot readily be seen.[13]

Brueggemann uses the term '(non) existence' to demonstrate how she seems not to feel fully alive in either world. In the shadow of the dominant groups of hearing and heterosexuality, the deaf and gay/lesbian groups seem to lose substance. To become visible, they need to assert themselves with a voice.

This process is hardly clear-cut. In an essay on the similarities between non-visible disabilities and femme lesbian identity, which is often excluded or ignored in the lesbian community, scholar Ellen Samuels suggests that the term 'coming out', or declaring one's disability or sexuality, needs to be contextual. It is not 'a static and singular event...an over-the-rainbow shift that divides one's life before and after the event'.[14] Rather, the decision to come out changes according to context, whether this is personal, professional or political. This context is particularly important for people with non-visible disabilities. Often it's assumed that, if a person looks like they can function well, then they cannot be disabled.

For many in the Deaf community, this visibility is achieved through sign language. For those who are deaf and do not sign, however, interactions with hearing people sometimes require a request for light by which to see a face, or to speak more slowly and clearly, all of which are awkward with someone you've only recently met. 'Coming out' also carries a risk of accusations of fraud.

To mitigate this, people with non-visible disabilities sometimes feel compelled to demonstrate a need for physical support, such as a cane for a blind person, even if that person can get by without it.[15] In my instance, I often flick back my hair to show my hearing aid as I tell people that I am deaf, knowing that I would hardly be believed otherwise. Doing this is problematic, however, for it confirms the stereotype that to be disabled one's disability must be obvious. There are no easy answers to these conundrums; it is up to the person with the disability to decide how and when they would like to reveal it.

~

In London, after years of either being heartbroken or married to my research, I had decided to resolve my singledom. Alex had faded incrementally from my consciousness, and my mind was once more my own. Late one Friday night after drinks with friends, the man who loved George Orwell, whom I met during my first days at the London Consortium, kissed me at Tottenham Court Road tube station. People swirled around us and his woollen coat brushed against my neck. I walked home in a daze.

Later, he apologised, 'I was pretty drunk.'

As always, I hid my disappointment.

In summer the pubs, which were always full, spilled people onto the pavements. They laughed as sunlight poured into their glasses of beer, while flowers frothed from window boxes. It was unexpectedly lovely.

It was also noisy, and I had to rely solely on lip-reading to communicate, which became impossible once a few drinks affected my concentration. At the Castle in Angel with Martine and Wojtek, I stopped listening and watched the faces of people around me instead.

'Can you see anyone you like, Jess?' Wojtek asked me.

I glanced again at the loud, laughing men. 'Not really. I wouldn't know how to talk to them, anyway.'

'You just look, catch his eye, and look away,' Martine explained. 'Then you look again and smile.'

'Oh God, I couldn't do that.' I'd need to explain that I was deaf. I shrank at the awkwardness that would inevitably follow.

Because I lost the part of my hearing that would respond substantially to lower pitches, I have to strain hard to hear men. Often I don't hear what they say at all, particularly if they have beards or moustaches and I can't see their lips.

When I was ten, my usual primary school teacher was away. We were placed in a class with older students whose teacher was a big, beefy man with the nickname Mr Growler. I didn't give him my FM because I was too afraid of approaching him.

'I have a question for you,' he said to the class, moving towards the windows on the far side of the room, where he leaned against the sill. With his back to the light, his face was in shadow and I couldn't lip-read him. I could also barely hear him from that distance. A few minutes passed and I began to panic; I didn't want to miss out. After a while I raised my hand and asked, 'What was the question?'

'I haven't asked the question,' he replied dryly. The room erupted into laughter and I looked down at my desk, my skin burning. From then on, I never asked anything unless I was sure of the context, particularly if I was speaking with a man.

In the pub, I reminded myself that I must be less guarded and that I must get over my fear of humiliation. But when I watched the faces of the men around me laughing and chatting, a pit opened in my stomach. What if they didn't accept me because of my deafness? The thought frightened me so much that I looked down at my drink to avoid catching anyone's eye.

Assuming that it would be less awkward than straining to hear in a noisy London pub, I decided to try internet dating. Oliver and I sat at the kitchen table, my fish tank burbling before us, to write my profile and select some photos.

On the weekend, I drank tea with Oliver in the garden and complained, 'I'm not getting any replies. They write me one line and I reply with several paragraphs and then I don't get anything back.'

'My God, Jess, you don't write paragraphs! At least, not at the beginning. You'll scare everyone off.'

I was crestfallen. 'I haven't been doing that right, then.'

Oliver made a strange noise. I looked up and saw he was trying not to laugh. I began laughing, too, even as I was dismayed at having failed, once more, to understand social rules.

When I did eventually meet a man, I didn't have much luck. I was too earnest, approaching everything the same way I did in an essay, although I enjoyed the outings to pubs and plays. At the Barbican I told my date that I needed to check for hearing equipment before we saw a play. He waited while I spoke to the people in the box office and picked up some headphones. I could hear some of the play, but not all. Halfway through, I missed a joke.

He noticed that I wasn't laughing. 'Did you catch that?'

I shook my head and he repeated it for me. I was touched.

The next few dates were lacklustre, and I became disheartened. The man, while kind and interesting, didn't want to persist.

'I need to finish my research,' I tell Oliver.

'I think you're using that as an excuse.'

'Probably. But my research makes me happier than internet dating.'

From their first meeting in 1899, Nancy provided Rosa with companionship, emotional nourishment, secretarial help and an outlet for her spiritual yearnings. They travelled during the winters, survived the London bombings of the First World War (described by Rosa in that first letter of hers I had read in the British Library) then, as their lives slowed, moved to Torquay to be closer to Maud.

Nancy died on 24 May 1927 from heart failure, emphysema and oedema, twenty-eight years after her and Rosa's first meeting.[16] Rosa's suffering upon the death of her friend was unbearable. Amid the tragedy of Maud's poorly treated mental illness and the premature death of Rosa's husband and all three of her sons (her youngest, Geoffrey, was gored by a rhino in a hunting accident in Rhodesia; Humphrey, as we have seen, was killed in a car crash in California; and Bulkley, her closest, who had struggled often with depression, shot himself when it became uncontrollable), Nancy had provided love, support and emotional nourishment.

To assuage her grief, Rosa tried to contact Nancy using a medium, Hester Dowden. The daughter of an Irish literary scholar, Dowden grew up with the literary elite of Dublin passing through her house, and claimed to have communicated with Francis Bacon, William Shakespeare and Oscar Wilde.[17] She published the words of the latter in 1923 as *Psychic Messages from Oscar Wilde*.

I imagine Rosa in Dowden's drawing room in 15 Cheyne Gardens in Chelsea. The London light, extraordinarily strong for a May afternoon, pours through the French windows. Rosa sits in an armchair, a red cushion supporting her lower back. The room is cluttered with cups and saucers, piles of shells, pieces of half-finished embroidery stretched over frames, a Pekinese that, unaccustomed to the heat, sits panting beneath the table. Opposite Rosa, Mrs Dowden, her greying hair softly waved, sits erect in her chair. A board, some foolscap paper and several sharpened pencils lie in her lap.[18]

Rosa's heart is beating too fast. She asks, 'May I try to reach her first?'

One of the cats stretches, blinking slowly against the sun.

'Of course, Mrs Praed,' Mrs Dowden smiles.

Rosa takes the board and pencil. She sits still, waiting. Her hand begins to produce marks and unintelligible letters, then it slows and stops. Rosa looks at the scribble, dismayed.

'Perhaps I shall try?' Mrs Dowden suggests gently.

Rosa nods and gives back the board.

When Mrs Dowden takes the pencil, the writing immediately becomes clear, firm and fast. Rosa fights to remain patient as the medium's hand moves swiftly across the page. After ten minutes of the scratching pencil, the dog's panting and the whirr of traffic beyond the windows, Rosa can stand it no longer. When Mrs Dowden's hand slows, she interrupts, even at the risk of breaking the medium's connection with Nancy.

'Might I know what she has said?'

Mrs Dowden gazes at her and Rosa is unsure as to whether the medium is still listening to the astral plane, or if she's back in the drawing room. Then she looks down at what she has written. 'My dear, dear, dear, I can't tell you what it has been to be without you. I have stood beside you hundreds of times – hundreds, but I can't get through the barrier.'[19] She pauses, swallowing. Rosa leans forward.

'My dearest, I have been with you constantly, in fact now you are on my plane as much as you are on your own. I came here and pressed for entrance, because I felt I must break the silence. Your loneliness has impressed us all so much, that we felt we must speak to you in words.'[20]

'Oh, at night,' Rosa says aloud, 'I have been overwhelmingly conscious of you. So much that it hurts, makes me cry.'[21]

Dowden continues, 'Your thoughts are so clear to me that it seems much less confusing than a conversation. The meaning of words is fuller than the words themselves. I actually hear you think of me.'[22]

This was a literary seduction. Rosa, desperate to be with Nancy once more, tried to draw her close through writing.

At the same time she was seeing Dowden, Rosa decided to rewrite *Nyria* the way she had always wanted to, with footnotes that verified the historical scenes Nancy had described under hypnosis. This way, Rosa could prove that, if the events actually happened as Nancy recalled them, then she and Rosa really were the current incarnations of Nyria and Valeria. And if this was true, then they would continue to reincarnate, and they would be together once more in the future.

Rosa contacted Nancy through Dowden and compiled notes on the incarnations of Nyria and her friend Valeria before and after their Roman lives. The first incarnation was 'some two or three hundred years after the submergence of Atlantis in about 9000 B.C.', continuing through to South America, North Africa and France, then manifesting as Nyria and Valeria.[23]

To prove that Nyria's story as narrated by Nancy was not fiction, but an actual case of reincarnation, Rosa employed Ralph Shirley, an occultist, author, director of the publishers William Rider & Son, and founder of the *Occult Review*, to verify all the details and incidents in the novel.[24] They worked intensely on the project for several hours a day, an extraordinary effort for a woman who was nearly eighty. Rosa's dedication illuminates the magnitude of her loss and her longing to be with Nancy once more.

Eventually, Rosa had a falling-out with Shirley because he was pedantic and immovable on some points. Rosa wrote to her half-sisters Ruth and Dorothy:

> I feel I *can't* go on working with him and shall try to hold him to his letter saying that if Nyria is wrong about Aemilia's death (the date) her story is a fabrication – but I am very much afraid he will not give it up – for his own sense would tell him that one flaw in more than 100 verifications does not make the psychological phenomenon the any less remarkable.[25]

Later, Rosa's publishers did not want Shirley to be on the contract and lawyers became involved. Rosa went to a session with Dowden for guidance and was counselled by the spirits not to stir the nest.[26] In 1931 Rosa published her historical notes, together with the original story, as *Soul of Nyria: The Memory of a Past Life in Ancient Rome.*

By using Shirley, Rosa imitated similar researchers, such as those who formed the Society for Psychical Research (SPR), who wanted to prove that supernatural phenomena were real. The SPR, which was formed in 1882, included Henry Sidgwick and his wife Eleanor, Frederic Myers, Edmund Gurney and Frank Podmore. The men had studied science at Oxford and Cambridge, and believed the scientific method could be applied to the supernatural to prove its existence. In 1886, Gurney, Podmore and Myers published *Phantasms of the Living*, which, through over seven hundred case studies of events such as telepathy, clairvoyance and hypnosis, attempted to provide a body of scientific evidence to support the existence of psychic phenomena. Rosa knew Myers, and in 1884 received an invitation from him to meet for lunch.[27] She also corresponded with William Crookes, who was elected a fellow of the Royal Society for scientists in 1863 and was president of the Society for Psychical Research from 1896 to 1899.

Crookes was a member of the Theosophical Society and when *Nyria* was published in 1904, Rosa sent him a copy. In response, Crookes wrote,

> I was very pleased to receive your letter, with the assurance that the introductory note was really a statement of fact. For myself I required no such assurance, but I am glad to be able to tell friends to whom I have recommended 'Nyria' that I have that assurance in your writing.[28]

This process of verifying the paranormal was old-fashioned by the 1930s, although spiritualism remained in vogue during and after the First World War because of heartbroken family, friends and lovers wanting to contact loved ones they had lost in the carnage. Rosa, who was isolated towards the end of her life due to infirmity, still held on to the character that had introduced and then bound her to Nancy, and that held out the promise of an eternal life together.

I sympathise with her. For all my reticence towards her because of what happened to Maud, I understand how terrible it is to be deprived of someone you love. Rosa had lost her husband, sons and daughter, at least the one that she had known. Nancy, who had made up for all this, was now gone, too.

In 1932, towards the very end of her life, Rosa wrote to her half-sisters Ruth and Dorothy, 'I cannot think that the deep love Nancy gave me – the one absolutely unselfish love I have been blessed in knowing – can count for nothing – no one – even my own children – ever loved me as she loved me – and could that mean nothingness?'[29]

I don't believe in reincarnation, but I am glad that Rosa's suffering and heartsickness finally ceased when she died of heart disease on 10 April 1935, eight years after Nancy.

~

In Brisbane, I sign up to more internet dating sites. Despite my distaste for dating, the romantic in me won't be quelled. On the profile I put together, I don't mention my deafness. I've read enough on social media feeds to know this would be akin to romantic suicide, though I do worry that I'm letting the side down by not challenging stereotypes of disability.

I skip over pictures of men with motorbikes, surfboards and utes, then come across a fresh-faced fellow with a nice smile. We start chatting and I agree to meet him for dinner. We exchange phone numbers in case something goes awry. The evening before we meet, my mobile, which I only use for texting, begins to ring. It's the fellow from the dating site.

My heart rate rockets during the staticky conversation, which is pocked with deep silences. After several minutes, in which I slowly work out that he's calling for a chat rather than to tell me of a change of plans, I make an excuse to hang up. Why had he called me when he couldn't carry the conversation?

I'm still rattled the next evening as I walk down Boundary Road in West End to the restaurant. When I meet him, I calm down. He's a small, unassuming guy who works in electronics, synchronising lights. I'm not attracted to him, but when I get home I write down some of his stories, which made me smile.

A while later, I meet a Scottish electrician in a café opposite Mowbray Park. He's open, friendly and, when I explain I'm deaf, makes an effort to speak clearly amid the clanging of cutlery.

Out of the blue, he asks, 'You don't have a ute, do you?'

'Ah, no.'

'And do you go camping?'

I thought it best to be honest. 'No. I don't like camping much.'

'Thank God for that! So many women I've met like driving round in utes, camping and shooting things. It's so nice to meet a lady.'

I smile, pleased.

This fellow seems appreciative of my writing. 'It's great that you're so devoted to what you do. I don't think I could get so passionate about fixing lifts!'

I wish that I could have liked him more. Regretfully, we part ways.

I had read fairytales: all Sleeping Beauty had to do was sleep for a century and a man fell in love with her. She didn't even have to speak to him. Despite my refashioning of this tale in my childhood stories, I assume that if men don't fall in love with me instantaneously then there's something I'm not doing right. I put it down to my deafness and poor social skills, but my friends keep telling me there's nothing wrong with my interactions with people.

Another offers the advice, 'If a man says something to you at the bar and you don't hear it, all you have to do is say, "Sorry, I'm deaf, what was that you said? Were you going to buy me a drink?"'

I shake my head. I have none of this friend's confidence.

'Maybe you're too picky.'

'Why shouldn't I be? I'm giving up my writing time for this person. They have to be worth it.'

'Just persist. Sometimes you need to have more than a few dates for it to work.'

These days, I'm perturbed that it mattered to me so much. I liked my own company and I didn't need a partner for emotional succour, but I missed sex and the comfort of a body at night. I was also, despite being a feminist, never able to rid myself of the fantasy that I had expressed in my writing and that had drawn me to Rosa's romantic novels: that I would be loved without reservation.

Rosa's romance *Lady Bridget in the Never-Never Land*, published in 1915, was her third-last novel. Her two protagonists, a flighty, excitable Englishwoman and a salt-of-the-earth Australian farmer are diametrically opposed in their personalities. Despite this, they are attracted to one another, and marry. Their relationship is abraded by the hardship of drought and Bridget's unfamiliarity with the harsh life of a farmer's wife. When she receives an unexpected inheritance, she leaves her husband. After a while apart, the couple swallow their pride, overcome their differences and reunite. The final line shows their transformation through love: 'And in that kiss, by the divine alchemy of true wedded love, all the past pride and bitterness were transmuted into a great abiding Peace.'[30]

I adored the promise in these novels of unconditional acceptance through love. I was convinced that if someone loved me, my disability would cease to matter. I should have realised the dissonance in my reading: that Rochester had to be burnt before he learned to love Jane Eyre, and that Rosa forced Maud to conform to the hearing world by learning to speak, rather than accepting her as she was; that she became so caught up with Nancy that she neglected her daughter.

A man sends me a request to meet. His profile picture doesn't attract me but he's an engineer. One of my flatmates in Surry Hills was an engineer and her humour appealed to me. With my friend's advice on persistence still echoing, I accept the man's offer. He might, I reason, be more interesting in the flesh.

That Sunday I walk over the Story Bridge to the Valley, hungover from dancing and drinking the night before, listening to music on an iPod. I hope the exercise will take the edge off my seediness, but when I reach the Valley mall and check the address where we agreed to meet, I realise it's the same place I'd been dancing in the night before.

The man sits at a table outside. I stretch out my hand in greeting, but his handshake is limp. I head into the bar and buy a drink. The floor is still sticky.

In the sun outside, we talk about the man's job. He describes how distressing it is to work for an intensive care unit in which architecture and health considerations make it impossible for mothers to be with their tiny premmie babies. I soften towards him. He talks largely about himself and asks nothing about my life, so I begin describing my books and writing. His face turns blank.

I walk back over the bridge. That alien feeling, which cloaked my shoulders when I sat beneath the jacaranda tree as a schoolgirl, now wraps me tighter. When I reach home, I open my laptop and delete my dating account.

Alex, who married while I was living in London, has moved to Brisbane. By emailing intermittently over the years, we have patched things into a friendship. I realised that I never wanted to lose contact with him, because he knew me so well. Once he called me 'a stubborn bitch who doesn't know how to lose' and I was chuffed.

We meet up for coffee now and then. When I see him at the door my heart lifts, but I never let it show. I accept that I'll always feel like this, but that I don't need to act on it. I complain to him about my dating disasters.

'It's hard for me to watch you going through this,' he says.

I'm furious. I think of the depression I endured and the years of work I put into getting over him. 'I processed all my feelings for you years ago.'

He stops emailing. I don't let it bother me.

As I ride my bicycle along the Brisbane River, the dank smell of mangroves rising from the water, my thoughts tend to Maud, who was taught to ride a bicycle when she was ten. Campbell arranged for her to leave her bicycle at the Trafalgar Cycling Club in Chelsea Square for repairs. This was just down the road from the Praeds' house in London at 75 Elm Park Gardens. In a letter to her aunt Dorothy when she was about twenty-one, Maud suggested that she was also able to ride in the square itself, as she wrote, 'There is a large track in the square by the club house with a smoothly mown lawn where lawn tennis or croquet can be played. I cannot ride through the traffic for fear of an accident.'[31] Maud's deafness would have meant she couldn't hear the carriages around her and was at risk of being knocked from her bike.

Maud must have longed to do so many things, but found herself unable to because of her deafness and, later, her mental illness. I have no doubt that she would have wondered whether she would find an admirer. After all, Rosa expected Maud to move among and socialise with hearing people. Maud, who enjoyed company, would have tried to learn their customs and social rules, which included courtship and marriage.

In her journal about her travels in Japan, Maud described a steep climb up a mountain with her mother and a friend. A 'coolie' 'held his arm round my waist in case I might fall over the dangerous gorge. What a strange feeling it was. Mrs Crosby was helped by a chivalrous coolie. She looked thankful because of her widowhood.'[32] Was the feeling strange because Maud was so unused to being touched by a man, or was it because of the precipitous gorge? Why did her next thought move to Mrs Crosby and her widowed state?

Was it the weight of social expectation that made her stomp up and down the corridor of her asylum several years later, shouting that 'she had got to marry Frank, she was going to marry Frank. Where was Frank?'[33] Did Maud think that if she married Frank

D'Arcy, she would be able to go home? Or was she, like many young women, simply wanting to share her body with someone?

I'm reminded of the film *Babel*, in which an accident connects four groups of people on three different continents: two young Moroccan goatherds, a vacationing American couple, a deaf Japanese teenager and her father, and a Mexican nanny who takes her young charges across a border without their parents' permission. In one scene Chieko, the deaf teenager, takes off her knickers beneath the table of a café and shows her vagina to a boy. Later, she attempts to seduce a police officer investigating her father. When this fails, she takes off her clothes and walks outside into the freezing Tokyo night to stand on the balcony of her father's apartment.

When I saw the naked girl in the film standing in the cold, I could imagine what she felt. The girl was calling for someone to caress her body, but she couldn't muster a conversation to get to that point.

At least, living one hundred years after Maud, I've been able to have flings without the opprobrium of a conservative society, as she could not. Nor, arguably, could her mother. Yet it is still so very difficult.

On a balmy Brisbane evening in September 2012, my second novel *Entitlement* is launched by a local writer, Kris Olsson. This is the first time I've met her, though we've exchanged emails. She is, I come to find, a beautiful, kind woman, gently incisive in her perspectives. We sit before the audience, Kris to my right so that I can hear her. The room is crowded with my friends. I wonder how I've gone from knowing just three people three years ago to this room full of friendly faces. Perhaps I'm more of an extroverted

White than I realise. Perhaps I simply perform differently, through words, the same way, if I reach back into my literary history, my relative Patrick White did.

Where I feel an affinity with him is not so much through his large canvases, thick with literary arabesques and sharp, wry humour, but rather through his sense of being an outsider, an artist and a homosexual in a farming family that was even more conservative than mine. Yet his family still supported him. His father gave him a stipend while he wrote his first novel in London, just as my parents had supported me through my writing degree at the University of Wollongong and again when I moved, broke, to Brisbane.

I recognised a long time ago that, even though my mother never expressed her love for me physically, she was always generous and supportive in practical ways. She tried to find me space and time to write if I needed it. Tonight she sits in the front row. Oliver, who has moved back to Sydney, is beside her. Bella, her husband and their kids are a few rows back. My father sits to the side so he can take photos.

'He looked,' a friend later tells me, 'as pleased as punch.'

During question time, my mother gives away the plot to the audience, most of whom haven't yet read the book. Then Kris comments in response to a question, 'By the time you reach your second or third book, you can see patterns forming.'

This strikes me like an arrow. From the moment of its conception, I knew *A Curious Intimacy* would be about a woman who had lost her baby and subsequently became unhinged. In an earlier short story, I followed in painstaking detail a mother's discovery of her child's cot death. At the heart of *Entitlement* was the loss of a brother.

My parents never spoke about Hamish. My mother, a stoic woman, accepted it and moved on. My father is a sensitive man; the sound of organs makes him want to weep. Perhaps he couldn't trust himself to bring it up. Instead, in that silence, their grief flowered in my writing.

A few days later, Oliver and I take our niece and nephew to the pool for their swimming lessons. While they're busy, we cross the grounds to the adults' pool to cool off. Oliver tells me about a dinner he'd had with a family friend the other evening. This friend had mentioned an ability to see and communicate with spirits. After dinner, Oliver asked him for a reading.

'What was it like?'

'Weird. It was as though he was looking over my shoulder, staring hard at something.'

'What was he seeing?'

'There was an old man in a hat standing by a clothesline, holding a dead rabbit, and another man in a kaftan with a beard.'

The images were nebulous and needed interpretation, a fitting to the frame of our family history.

'Then he said to me, "Was there anything else you wanted to ask?"'

Oliver must have looked nervous, for our friend said, 'Everyone's usually got something they want to ask.'

'Well, there is. There was another White, in between my sisters, but he died when he was eight months old. I was wondering, can you see him there?'

'Yes, I can. He's fine, he's happy, and he's holding your mum's heart.'

Unexpectedly, my eyes become hot with tears and I'm grateful for my sunglasses. Brisbane is at the tail end of a decade-long drought and the grass beneath my feet is so dry it's white.

A few months later, I meet Donna for lunch at the trendy Sixes and Sevens bar in New Farm. We sit in a quiet part of the room and catch up on each other's work. I'm unwell and in the middle of writing a particularly difficult essay, and I feel low. Somehow, in response to Donna's reference to the loss of her son, I explain that my mother had also lost her child. To my alarm, I begin weeping. I apologise and Donna waves it away.

'Deaf children,' she says, 'are alert and observant. They absorb all that they can see and sense, even when that happens subliminally.'

When I was six, visiting a dinosaurs exhibition at the Australian Museum in Sydney on our annual holiday, someone picked the lock of our red Commodore and drove it away. Dad went off to find the cops. We waited with Mum under a tree in Hyde Park, sitting in the grass with our books, while she remained standing. My shoulder touched her calf.

'Will we get the car back, Mum?' I craned my head to look at her.

'I don't know, darling. Just read your book.'

Dutifully, I opened my colouring-in book on dinosaurs and scratched inside a T-Rex with a green pencil. I sensed my mother's anxiety in the stiffness of her legs as she looked out for my father.

The police found the car a few days later. The crims had taken our cassettes, but left a boomerang in their place. When we arrived back at the farm, Dad took us into the paddocks to show us how it worked.

I wonder if telepathy is no more than the ability to decode body language and intuit what someone is thinking, the way I could feel my mother's stress travelling down her body into mine. The term 'telepathy' was coined by Frederic Myers in 1882 and means 'to feel at a distance'. In his introduction to *Phantasms of the Living*, his colleague from the Society for Psychical Research, Frank Podmore, defined the term as 'all classes of cases where there is reason to suppose that the mind of one human being has affected the mind of another, without speech uttered, or word written, or sign made'.[34] It offered the opportunity to be inside another's mind, so that every thought and feeling was understood immediately, without an intermediary.

Has deafness made me able to feel things at a distance? I'm hypersensitive to discomfort in conversations or social situations. When I upset someone, I feel their distress as if it were my own. If I'm told about a break-up, or someone stepping on broken glass, I wince.

Once, at the British Library, I stopped at the issue desk to collect a book, but I couldn't hear the elderly staff member speaking to me.

'I'm sorry,' I said, 'but I'm deaf and I can't hear you very well. Could you please repeat what you said?'

The man cupped his hands around my mouth and shouted at me. Mute with shock, I collected my book and walked away.

When I relayed this conversation to my parents on the phone that weekend, Dad said, 'You're too sensitive.' This made me feel worse. I have to be sensitive so that I pick up cues I might miss because I can't hear them.

Once again, deafness is a *pharmakon*, a poison and a cure. It makes me receptive enough to body language and mannerisms to keep up in a conversation, but it also makes me porous, more susceptible to hurt, more alert to others' mourning and grief.

~

Through a library talk to promote *Entitlement*, I meet a teacher who works with deaf children. She invites me to give a talk at a conference for teachers for the deaf. I can't agree fast enough.

Mr Tony, who'd visited me in preschool, was my first support teacher. He took me for a lesson once a week. For this I used a separate exercise book from my schoolbooks. It was red with a picture of Snoopy cut out and glued on the front. Mr Tony taught me prepositions by drawing a picture in my book of a table with an open drawer. He wrote around it, in tiny writing, *in*, *on* and *under*.

One afternoon, as we walked around the playground watching the set-up for a fundraising day organised by the pupils, Mr Tony took me to a stand. On it rested a tray of sand garnished with pebbles, a small plastic treasure chest and a pile of toothpicks topped with paper flags.

'It's a scavenger hunt,' he explained. 'You put your flag where you think the treasure is and the person closest wins. The treasure's over here.' He pointed to the top left corner of the tray.

The next day, among children swishing their hands through buckets of lucky dips, crouching in a tent made of sheets to have their palms read, or paying twenty cents to guess which of the school's red-haired identical twins was which, I wandered to the treasure hunt. I handed over my coin and picked up a flag. It hovered over the sand while I debated the ethics of placing my toothpick where I knew the treasure to be. I desperately wanted the prize: textas and crayons nestled in a clear plastic satchel that shone in the light. But Mr Tony would find out and he would know that I had cheated. With a sigh, I placed my flag further away from the treasure and won third prize.

Mrs Matthews, who replaced Mr Tony when I began Year Three, taught me to tell the time, answered any questions I had about schoolwork or classmates, and helped with my speech.

'Oliver and I found a dead ibith in the paddock.'

'Ibissss. Tuck your tongue behind your front teeth when you say "s". Ibis.'

Eventually, with her help and the repeated work of my parents, any trace of an impediment was removed from my speech, although the trained ears of speech therapists can still find the lisp lurking in some words and, my parents tell me, on rare occasions I sound flat.

My teachers never made me feel stigmatised. Rather, I revelled in the extra attention and activities. I reasoned that I was special because of my disability. Mrs Matthews's stickers, her praise for my stories, the quiet comfort of her presence, boosted my confidence. If, during my teens, I'd been able to hold onto this sense, I might not have derailed into an eating disorder.

Six months after meeting with the teachers for the deaf, I stride into the Convention Centre in South Brisbane. I catch the lift upstairs, stepping into a crowd of people milling on a balcony. I take a glass of champagne from a passing waiter and gaze around. Some people are speaking and some are signing, their hands elegant in the pale, artificial light.

I'm reminded of a man who came to clean my carpet a few months before. As he was bald, his hearing aids were obvious. He explained the process of cleaning the carpet, then added, 'By the way, I'm deaf. If I have my back to you, I probably won't hear you.'

'I noticed. I'm deaf, too.' I lifted my hair to show him my hearing aid and his face lit up. I explained I'd had meningitis. He had been born deaf and went to Tamworth High School. At the school, he and his deaf friends had devised their own home signs for talking to one another.

'How many of you were there?' I asked.

'Five or six.'

I was astonished there could be so many deaf kids in one school. I'd barely met any deaf people and certainly none at school. I felt another sting of envy: he'd had a group to keep him safe and I had been irrevocably, coldly, alone. His mention of their own language didn't surprise me, though. It would have been easier for his deaf friends to communicate in sign, as it is for most deaf people.

Mr Tony taught me fingerspelling, which is spelling each letter of the alphabet. It's used in sign language when people want to spell out their name, or a proper noun. He had also taught me, and the children in my class, a few signs. In Year Two, I sat in the front row so I could hear. I usually heard or saw the teacher calling my name, but the boy next to me still liked to touch my arm and stroke his cheek with a forefinger to make the sign for 'teacher'.

Mum bought me a picture book with illustrations of signs, titled *Arabella, the Smallest Girl in the World.* Oliver and I pored over it, teaching ourselves to tell the story in sign. Aside from this, and the few dirty words that Oliver's best friend, a speech therapist, taught me a few years ago, I've had no experience with sign language. I know I ought to do something about this, and make a mental note to look up sign language classes.

At the conference for these teachers of deaf children, I'm mesmerised by their fast and fluid hands. I sip my glass of bubbles, watching them, until the conference organisers find me. Half an hour later I'm speaking at a podium, a translator signing beside me. I talk about how important my teachers had been and how my experiences of being deaf set me on the path to becoming a writer. I tell my stories about Mr Tony, then Mrs Matthews and the marijuana plants.

When I finish, the audience claps. Some shake their hands in the air, the sign for clapping in sign language. I'm stunned by the applause and, afterwards, by people's warmth as I sell copies of *Entitlement*. It's as though a door has opened and I can see the firelight of a hearth flickering within.

~

As the days heat, Oliver comes to Brisbane for another visit. I have moved out of Bella's into an apartment in East Brisbane, which isn't far away. Oliver and I round up our niece and nephew for a trip to the beach at South Bank.

'Watch out for paedophiles,' Bella says, smearing green sunscreen onto the children's faces. 'I'm sure they hang out there.'

'Okay.' Oliver is nonplussed.

I go with them, but I don't swim. Not because of paedophiles but because the water is full of kiddy wee. I sit on the grassy bank, reading. Besides, Oliver has much more of a rapport with the children. Looking up from my book and watching them, I marvel at their confident splashing in the water.

On a holiday in New Zealand when I was twenty, Mum and I visited Hanmer Springs, a series of hot pools north of Christchurch. In the warm water, I wedged my back against a rough piece of rock and watched a little boy kick past in his circular floatie, as happy as a puppy left to romp in the grass. Over half of his face stretched a rosy birthmark, as though a sheet of melting plastic had wrapped across his cheek and burnt him. Watching him floating around, his face split by a smile, I couldn't help but smile in return. He was oblivious to the stain on his face, for which, one day, he might be victimised.

I hoped he wouldn't. I hoped he'd be wrapped in a soft, woollen blanket of acceptance, as I had been at the hospital when I had my tonsils out. At school, under the guidance of my teacher, every child in my class made a *Get Well Soon Jessica* card, decorated with awkwardly cut-out circles and coloured in with streaky pencils. I still have the wad of cards, wrapped in a plastic bag.

People also dropped by the hospital with gifts for me. When it was time to go, I noticed that there was one more, still wrapped and left on the bedside table. I sensed that I wasn't supposed to touch it, but reasoned that I could justify unwrapping it by saying that I had assumed it was for me, as every other gift had been. As I peeled off the paper, I discovered a jar full of boiled sweets.

My mother returned, saw the jar and scolded me. 'Jessica! That was for the nurses, not you.' She disappeared, returned with some Sellotape and patched up the wrapping.

I felt small and mean in my thin nightie, and decided not to justify myself.

This didn't stop me, on our return home, from taking out all the presents I'd been given and lining them up on the table on the verandah. I found Oliver watching television, mouth agape, and dragged him away from the screen.

'Look,' I said, showing him the presents on the table. 'Look how much everyone loves me.'

That winter at a party, I meet an engineer. I like his face, framed with square glasses, and his jokes. My laughter carries over the balcony into the Brisbane night. We exchange email addresses.

Over the next few months, I find him refreshingly frank in his affections, but occasionally he drops the phrase, 'not looking for anything long term'. A friend mentions he's recently broken up with his girlfriend. He invites me to a ball for engineering students at which he's been invited to speak. I wear a long, silk dress that swishes when I gather it up to step into the cab.

When the cab driver dithers over the address, the engineer snaps, 'Look, mate, just go and we'll work it out.'

The sharpness in his voice unsettles me.

At the ball, he's uncomfortable with dancing, so I chat to the man sitting next to me in an interminable conversation that I can't hear because the music is so loud. I learned a long time ago that a smile and nod in the right places is enough to make a man think you're interested. I wish I had enough courage to tell him to speak up, but the habit of hiding my deafness is too deeply ingrained. Also, the effort involved would kill his conversation.

The engineer wants to go clubbing with the students afterwards but I'm worn out from trying to hear. Reluctantly, he comes home with me.

I stay at Bella's for a few days to dogsit her cocker spaniels while she's on holidays with her family. Bentley was my running companion the year I lived at her house. Whenever I visit he recognises me and turns inside out with pleasure. The other dog is blind, her eyes having been taken out when her retinas dislodged. Oliver's name for her is 'Tiresias'.

I ask the engineer if he wants to go to South Bank to see some fireworks, but instead he comes around to the house. We sit on the day bed on the verandah, smoke from a mosquito coil at our feet drifting into the air.

'I don't think this is working,' he begins.

'What? Why not?'

'I travel a lot.'

'That doesn't bother me.'

After a few minutes, I work out that these glib phrases are get-out-of-jail-free cards. I draw my knees up to the couch and wrap my arms around them, protecting myself, the way I have since I was small. 'Just leave.'

Eventually, he does. My sobbing carries through the still, suburban night. Bentley inches forwards and licks my toes.

Entitlement doesn't sell as well as *A Curious Intimacy*. The mechanism, embedded since childhood, of relying on academic and literary success to compensate for what I perceive as inadequacy, is broken. I should recognise the pattern from my time in London: continual crying, bone-deep exhaustion and working constantly to make up for a pervasive sense of defeat. But where *A Curious Intimacy* remedied my sadness in London, this time there is no reprieve. The familiar sense of failure, of sitting alone on a bench, unable to participate, envelops me.

Once again, I try to get outside to stymie my depression, regardless of my tiredness. I attend a lecture arranged by a literary journal at the State Library of Queensland. The loop system in the lecture theatre isn't loud enough and the frustration of trying to hear the speakers brings me to tears. I can't hold back my bitterness, either, that on the stage I'm watching a row of successful writers and I am still unknown.

I should be reminding myself that I have published two novels and won scholarships. I should be repeating to myself my own words from many years before in the conversation with the study abroad interviewer in Wollongong: *Writing is a craft. It takes a long time to become good at it.* I should be recalling that I have been brave enough to face the thing that terrified me most: stepping onto a plane and leaving my family for a year in a foreign country. But depression has narrowed my vision and made it hard to gain perspective. I feel that writing, so long my comfort and confidante, has betrayed me.

I now know, several years after the novel was born into the world, that sometimes books don't resonate, for whatever confluence of reasons. I also didn't have a network of writers to bolster me. Ever slow with my socialising, it took me a long time to connect with and become friends with other writers in Brisbane. Had I had writer friends, they would likely have told me that the emotions I experienced, watching those writers on the stage, was something that many emerging writers feel. Instead, my isolation – as it had when I was small and my cousins and siblings moved away – made me feel the loss of the book's success keenly.

After the talk at the State Library, there's a drinks reception on the adjoining terrace. It's a lovely area, exposed to the cool evening air, but for a deaf person it's a nightmare: all of the surfaces are tiled, making sound reverberate, and my hearing aid amplifies everything. I take it out and rely on lip-reading. Donna's in the crowd, and she introduces me to other writers. I use the last vestiges of my energy to concentrate on what they're saying.

When Donna leaves, I realise I'll be left among strangers. I can't bear it and leave with her.

As we walk down the steps, she asks, 'How are you?'

'I'm stressed,' I blurt. I explain the broken relationship, my inability to stop working and relax.

'You sound like you've got a bit of anxiety. Maybe you should go and see someone?'

I hug Donna goodbye and catch the bus home. When I get off at my stop and walk up the dark street overhung by fig trees, I start crying and can't stop for three days.

I ask Mum for some money to see a psychologist. She emails in response, *Of course. We believe in you implicitly and where you are going.*

I smile, tiredly, at this pinprick of light.

In a doctor's surgery I explain, once again, about my deafness, the anorexia, my workaholism, the demands I place upon myself to succeed.

'You're working yourself to death!' the psychologist exclaims.

I shrug.

I Skype Oliver. 'I need a break. Will you come to far north Queensland with me? I can do some research for my next book while I'm there.'

'Sure.'

A few weeks later, I meet him at the airport in Townsville. We pick up a hire car and drive to Cardwell, a pretty town where we stop to look at the ocean. At the lookout over the beach, a girl stands next to us with her dog, also admiring the view.

'His name's Atticus,' she introduces him. 'Shake.' The dog lifts his paw. 'Roll over.' He lies down and shows his tummy. Oliver and I laugh. We walk along the beach as the light fades.

'What about the crocodiles? What if they run in from the sea and eat us?'

'It's not the season for them, Jess.'

I make sure Oliver is closer to the water than I am.

At Atherton we investigate an Art Deco pub and an old Chinese joss house, and swim in crater lakes with children and small turtles. We walk through Mount Hypipamee National Park and encounter a very angry cassowary that charges at me. I turn, expecting the worst, and find that Oliver is standing it down, his hand outstretched, hissing at it. The cassowary, seeing that Oliver is taller than him and making aggressive noises, figures he is not worth the fight. It walks away, leaving us shaken.

We snorkel off the reef near Cape Tribulation, stingrays and gigantic angelfish drifting beneath us. We spend the last few days at Trinity Beach, north of Cairns. As we sit in the sand, Oliver reads and I watch the crests of waves foaming and dissolving as they run into the shore. I think about the sessions with the psychologist that I've had over the past few weeks.

I know that all my rosettes for drawing and painting, my Eisteddfod trophies for piano, my academic transcripts full of high distinctions, my scholarships, my novels, my ability to speak so well that no one can tell I'm deaf, are a way of compensating for my disability. Part of it is also stubbornness: when someone tells me I can't do something, I go out of my way to prove them wrong. Another part of it is the compulsiveness of a perfectionist always trying to get things right. But the psychologist, an astute woman, has suggested a more subliminal reason for my constant and debilitating exertions. She thinks it might be to do with my older brother's death.

Somehow, being that quiet, watchful little girl, I had absorbed my mother's grief into myself. I worked hard for accolades not only because I liked the rewards, but because I wanted to shine with brilliance. That way, I could make up for everything my mother lost when her son died. Especially because, on that dark night in the hospital in Tamworth, she nearly lost me, too.

I discussed this with Mum not long ago, when she was in Brisbane and staying with Bella. 'This is not how I saw Hamish's death,' she said over a glass of wine on the verandah, 'but I can understand how you might arrive at that interpretation.'

I had the sense she wanted to say more but, after years of keeping my feelings to myself, I couldn't continue the conversation. We'll always be like this, two continental plates rubbing against one another, grit and salt mixing in our attempts to communicate. My mother cannot help the way she was put together, with a tremendous sense of responsibility for other people and a pragmatism that never lets emotion get in the way of anything, just as I cannot help the way my deafness, sensitivity and pride shaped me. But my mother still left me with a gift.

On an already hot Brisbane morning, my hearing aid turned off against the man mowing the lawns outside, my pen runs out of ink. I riffle for a new one in the box of stationery and paper I keep beside my desk and come across the orange National Australia Bank notebook I used as a diary when I was ten. On Tuesday 17 May 1988, I wrote, 'I worked on my social science and my spelling. I had to cross out some beautiful words which mum gave me. I couldn't bear to part with them. They held my mother's love.'

Where did this come from? Was I really so precocious at ten? Or was I simply less guarded? At that age, my head would turn like a sunflower whenever my mother entered a room. Once on the school bus, which had just pulled away from the school gates, I caught sight of our car parked at the kerb. I grabbed my bag and fled down the aisle.

'Stop!' I told the bus driver. 'My mum's across the road, she's come to pick me up!'

He opened the bus doors, cautioning me to watch out for cars, and I belted down the street. 'Hi, Mum!'

She frowned when she saw me. 'What're you doing here?'

I stopped running, realising that I didn't have any music lessons that day and that she wasn't there to pick me up. She must have just been in town doing errands. I didn't know what to say; I couldn't explain my mad delight on seeing her.

'Get in. I was going to do some jobs but we'll just go home.'

I was guilty that I had ruined her afternoon, but secretly pleased that I had her to myself for the whole car trip home.

If my mother gave me words, my father showed me the determination and ingenuity I needed to become a writer. When I was eight he decided he wanted some guineafowl for the chookyard because he liked their speckled feathers. From a neighbouring farmer he bought some guineafowl eggs and an old, circular incubator with six small holes. He placed the eggs in the holes, plugged the incubator into the wall of his studio, and turned the blow heater towards it.

At the same time, it transpired that the wife of a farmer who lived down the road had guineafowl living in her oak tree.

'If you can catch them, you can have them,' she said to Dad.

Oliver and I pulled on woollen beanies and gloves, and drove with Dad in the old Wolseley to the farmer's house. The oak tree was huge, arching over the back lawn. I had no idea how my father, armed with a spotlight and a long handheld net, was going to catch the birds.

He didn't.

'Never mind, kids,' he said after a spate of vicious swearing out of earshot of the farmer's wife. 'We've still got the eggs in the incubator.'

Not wanting to cook the chicks, he cracked three of the eggs open too soon, revealing a bloody mess of mucus and feathers. The remaining three hatched into chicks. He built a cage for them, lined it with chicken wire and made a small hessian tent at the end so they could keep warm.

One afternoon, as he mended a piece of machinery at the outdoor table by the cage, I joined him. The birds were half-grown, slightly bigger than my cupped hands, and sped sleekly from one end of the cage to the other. They seemed eerily intent, at least compared to chickens.

My father paused in his work, watching them, too. 'Look at that, Jess. It just goes to show there's no such word as "can't". If you really put your mind to something, you'll achieve it.'

I believed my father. His words took me to America and England, and meant I never gave up on trying to make it into print. I believe him still, but I also understand now that my determination has a huge emotional and physical cost. People might read my story and think it's inspiring. If they do, they should remember the disability activist Stella Young, who coined the term 'inspiration porn'. People with disabilities aren't put on earth to inspire other people; we're just trying to get on with our day in a world that isn't designed for us.

~

At my desk with the view of the palm trees and blue sky, I put the failure of *Entitlement* behind me and continue to write. Year after year, I apply for funding from the Australia Council for the Arts. At last, at the end of 2014, I'm successful in winning a two-month residency to write in a studio in Trastevere in Rome.

One morning, a few weeks into my stay, I walk from the studio to the nearby Botanical Gardens. Weak winter light falls through the oaks and their yellow leaves spiral to the ground. These leaves make no audible sound, although a person with all their hearing might hear them scratch lightly against the gravel. Yet, as my eye follows the arc of each leaf as it spirals down, I hear the sound of its descent in my head.

This process, known as 'auditory closure', is the ability to use contextual clues to work out pieces of an auditory signal that are missing. I've had a lifetime of practice in decoding the sounds I don't hear. If I only grasp part of a sentence, for example, I reach quickly for words and fit and discard them until the phrase makes sense. I'm not unique in using this technique. Donna, in her memoir, describes lip-reading as 'an art rather than a science'. She elaborates, 'I don't actually see or read every single syllable enunciated to me. I spend much energy guessing what is being said by filling in any missing information by drawing on the circumstances of the conversation.'[35] This practice becomes so familiar that partly deaf people extrapolate it to situations in which we can't hear at all.

While swimming with a friend, Donna had assumed she could hear, however faintly, the vowels in his voice without her hearing aid. However, when she thought about it, she realised she couldn't hear anything. Rather, as she writes, 'I had tricked even myself because I am so proficient at lip-reading, and because I know what his voice sounds like when I wear my hearing aids.'[36] Context is essential at these moments, as is the capacity to automatically fit words into a phrase until it makes sense.

Like Donna and rhetorician Brenda Jo Brueggemann, I rely on information I derive from tone or body language. A sentence will rise at the end if it's a question, a person's eyes will convey if they're happy, lying or troubled, while the restless beat of hands against a body or a man plucking at his suddenly tight collar might indicate apprehension or nervousness. Each moment is contextual, however, and only gathers meaning when taken as a whole.

This approach isn't foolproof. When I taught a class in English literature at the university in Brisbane, I turned around from writing 'fierce' on the whiteboard to rows of puzzled faces.

'I've heard the wrong thing, haven't I? Did you say "fierce" or "peace"?'

'Peace!'

'This is why I'm a creative writer,' I joked. 'I'm good at making things up.'

I turned and rubbed out *fierce*, replacing it with *peace*, hiding my old disquiet at having failed in the charade of hearing.

I walk out of the gardens and through the cobbled streets of Trastevere, heading for the Tiber River. The trees are bare and spindly. Together with the overcast sky and grey river, the atmosphere is melancholic. I don't mind it, as I did in London. The Mediterranean winter is mild, at least this December, although I've had to buy a new coat because after years in Brisbane I'd tossed out the ones from London. On sunny days the light falls delicately and it's nice to be in Rome without the summer rush of tourists.

I follow the curve of the river then cross Ponte Sublicio, heading for the markets at Testaccio. I buy fruit and flowers, using as few Italian words as possible, as I can't tell if I'm pronouncing them correctly. I like this area. Young people mill about and street art stretches up the sides of brick buildings. I cross another bridge, Ponte Testaccio, then head back to the studio where I'm staying.

Making meaning out of fragments of sound is relentless work, but it's also inherently creative. Many artists have found that disability engenders creativity. French composer Maurice Ravel's *Concerto for the Left Hand* was commissioned in 1930 by the pianist Paul Wittgenstein, who lost his right arm during the First World War. Composers such as Brahms, Saint-Saëns, Strauss, Prokofiev and Bartók created works for the left hand to showcase or strengthen it. Less well known is that these works were commissioned by pianists who had lost the use of one hand through repetitive strain injury or arthritis. Concertos like Ravel's show how disability forces people to think laterally and become adept in other ways. It liberates them from the traditional terms for composition.[37]

Liberation. It's not a word many would pair with disability. Yet it's one that works. For a long time I pitied myself because I could only stand on the fringes of conversations, unable to hear enough to join in, thinking that the people around me didn't care because they knew I was deaf and yet never included me. Like a ghost, I was deprived of a place to settle, as I belonged neither to the hearing nor the deaf world. If I tried to speak and claim my presence, I was sometimes laughed at or criticised for speaking out of turn, or for not speaking in the right way.

Yet is being a ghost so entirely impoverishing? Does not a ghost, in failing to belong, in travelling between worlds, in being forced to question and readjust, have a sensibility that is eerier, richer, more unearthly and extraordinary? Does not trying to reach another world make us more creative, more receptive to things that other people don't realise are there?

I stopped pitying myself when I realised that deafness was also a cure: it led me to writing and it helped me to become good at my craft. Being unable to participate with ease in conversations, for example, means I observe people instead, gathering details of their clothes, stance, facial hair and expressions for character descriptions. Having lost most of one sense, my others have become stronger, so I pay attention to textures, smells and visual details such as colour and light, using them to set my scenes. Disability forces me to solve problems, to think laterally, and to see and listen for the voices that others overlook.

Inside the apartment, I switch the kettle on, fretting over the lime deposits inside it. While the water heats, I head outside to the terrace lined with pot plants. The sun is setting over the city, the dusk of pale pink and purple enriching the terracotta roofs and the Vatican's dome.

There is also something in partial deafness, in moving between worlds, that nudges me towards the creation of story. Like the little girl who pestered her mother to piece together words on the camel-hair carpet, I want to learn, to be exposed to new sensations, to be unsettled and challenged, because this is how stories form.

Or do the stories find us? Without Rosa, I would not have found Maud, and without Maud, I would not have found the deaf part of myself that, for so long, had remained shadowy and unseen.

Some writers have a bible by their side as they work, a text to which they can refer when they get stuck. Mine is Margaret Atwood's *Negotiating with the Dead: A Writer on Writing*. Atwood muses that there are two selves that make up a writer: one who eats breakfast, goes shopping for groceries and walks the dog; and 'that other, more shadowy and altogether more equivocal personage who shares the same body, and who, when no one is looking, takes it over and uses it to commit the actual writing'.[38] This other self travels to the Underworld to talk to the dead, take their stories, and enlarge upon them for their readers. Atwood continues:

> All writers must go from now to once upon a time; all must go from here to there; all must descend to where the stories are kept...The dead may guard the treasure, but it's useless treasure unless it can be brought back into the land of the living and allowed to enter time once more – which means to enter the realm of the audience, the realm of the readers, the realm of change.[39]

My movement between temporalities, struggling to find words in the present and matching them with those in the past, mirrors Atwood's description of moving from the present to the past and back again to create meaning. The writer steals or recovers the stories from the dead and, as the everyday person who walks their dog, crafts them into something readable, just as I take what I have heard and fashion it into something that makes sense.

Atwood's realm of the dead can be interpreted as the writer's subconscious. In my subconscious is my parents' pool of grief, which wells into my writing. There's also my loneliness, my sense of shame and inadequacy, my receptiveness to the way people such as Maud have been damaged. It's a dark, desolate place. It's also the source from which I draw when I sit at my desk each day, the place where I talk to the dead, and take their stories into sunshine and clear air.

~

Back in Brisbane, I continue working on the story of Rosa and Maud, trying to find a shape that will hold our voices. In between my part-time jobs as a research assistant and sessional academic at the university, it is several years before I have something resembling a manuscript. I give it to my family to read. A few weeks later, I pedal down the road for a glass of wine with my sister. Bentley bowls me over when I open the gate.

We sit on Bella's verandah, a bottle of sauvignon blanc between us, crickets chirping in the grass, possums scuttling over the roof.

'Is this book a cry for help?' she asks me.

'No,' I frown. 'I don't need help. I've sorted everything out now.'

I have, by this stage, been living in Brisbane for nearly a decade. I have firm friends and I'm part of a literary network. I feel woven into the fabric of a place in a way I haven't experienced since I was a child on the farm.

'Why have you written it, then?'

'I'm tired of being taken for granted. I want people to know how hard I've worked – and how hard most people with disabilities have to work – to get where I am. I want them to hear Maud's voice and to know that, although things are much better, deaf people are still expected to act like hearing people. I want them to see how difficult it still is, when it shouldn't be. We're in the twenty-first century; it's not that hard to fix a loop system and make sure that it's working.'

Bentley clatters down the verandah stairs, barking at a possum in the garden. We refill our glasses. What I don't add is that I couldn't have said any of this without putting it into writing.

A few hours later, I pedal the few blocks back to my apartment, keeping to the footpath because, as for Maud, it's too dangerous for me to cycle on the road. I recall an exchange I had with a deaf woman at a conference for artists with disability in Sydney a few years ago.

It was the first time I'd used a translator. She stood next to me, signing my words and speaking those of the deaf woman who was talking to me. Out of habit, I turned to the translator to lip-read her.

'Don't look at me!' the translator snapped. 'Look at the person you're talking to.'

I apologised and turned to the woman who was deaf, even though it meant I had to strain to listen to the translator, who was repeating the woman's question.

'Do you identify as hearing or as deaf?'

I felt awkward, as if she was trying to flush me out, and thought about what to say. 'Probably as hearing. That was how I was raised.'

'Yes, that's what I thought.'

I was resentful that I had been asked this at all: did it really matter how I identified myself? Why could I not be both hearing and deaf, if this was what I was? And why was I being judged for the way I'd been brought up? In a way, it was no different from being raised Jewish or French.

After the conference, when I thought on this some more, my discontent flared into fury. The woman's question made me feel like a failure as a deaf person, as if I was an imposter at that conference because I could hear too well. Yet to say that I was hearing invalidated the loneliness, tiredness and strain I had experienced on account of being deaf. I was frustrated that I was expected to be either hearing or deaf, when I was neither.

Back at my apartment, I put my bike away in the laundry. Upstairs, my fish tank glows in the darkness, the fish butting the surface of the water for food. I resist turning on the light so I can watch them. Out the window, the palm tree makes a serrated silhouette.

I delved into the underworld through Rosa's words and discovered a woman who used writing to eclipse the distance from Australia and express her enduring love for Nancy. Then I found her daughter, who showed me the terrible history and impact of oralism. Without Rosa, and without Maud, I would never have found myself: a partly deaf, partly hearing woman who travels between worlds, and whose travelling made her a writer.

Epilogue

Grabbing Stars

On a summer evening that curls around my calves, I pull on a red frock and slip my feet into stilettos. I catch the bus to meet my friend Evie at Chinatown in the Valley. We sit outside a cheap restaurant on unsteady aluminium chairs, drinking white wine. After dinner, Evie checks her phone.

'Some friends of mine are playing in a band down the road. We can go and listen to them, if you like?'

I hesitate. 'It might be too noisy for me.'

'That's fine. We can go and see what it's like, and if it's too hard for you we can go somewhere else.'

We wander down to Alhambra. Outside, one of her friends is waiting for us. He's dark-haired and wears a white T-shirt and jeans. In my heels, I'm almost the same height as him. His name is Bruce. I shake his hand – his grip is firm – and we head inside the bar. The music pounds. Bruce asks me what I want to drink. I can't decide. I detest beer, it isn't the place for a civilised glass of wine, and it's too early in the night for spirits. The music is so loud it presses against me. I'm disorientated.

'Come on.' Bruce throws his arm around me and guides me to the bar, which gives me enough time to make a decision.

'I'll have a cider.'

With our drinks, we follow Evie outside to a tiny, paved courtyard. I take my hearing aid out so I can have a conversation. If I keep it in, it will magnify the music and drive me mad.

I hear about thirty per cent of what Bruce is saying and half of that is through lip-reading. He's studying philosophy at university; before that he'd been an ecologist. I tell him about the new fiction book I'm writing on oceans and climate change. He describes diving in Fiji. We discuss Campbell Newman, the newly elected premier, and his destructive environmental policies, and his destruction of everything, really. At some point I explain to Bruce that I'm deaf. I drink glass after glass of cider.

Eventually the lip-reading gets too hard, as it does when I'm drunk and my concentration is affected.

'I want to dance.'

Bruce follows me inside. Covertly, I watch him. His dancing isn't too bad.

I can only hear some of the melody against a blur of background noise, but I find the beat immediately.

I'd never have imagined, while stepping nervously to the music from a cassette with Mrs Matthews in the hall of Boggabri Primary School, how much I would come to love dancing, the feel of my body snapping to a rhythm. It reminds me of running on the farm, air touching my arms. When I move, joy wells and bubbles in my blood.

A song comes on with a slow beat buried beneath the bass, and I stop. 'I can't feel the beat.' This is unusual.

Bruce steps closer and clasps my forearm, tapping it out. I find the rhythm and start again. When he isn't looking, I glance at him. No other man has been smart enough to work out so quickly how to help me when I can't hear. Nor has a man been so uninhibited that he touches me in a way that isn't a drunken pass.

Bruce catches my eye and smiles.

A few hours later, we tumble onto the street. Heat rises from the pavement.

'Where would you like to go next?' Evie asks. 'Where's the place that you would most like to go to in the whole world?'

I brighten. 'The Bowery!'

We sidle towards the 1920s bootleggers' bar. I concentrate on the footpath, as my balance is worse when I'm drunk. I had once, after a boozy fundraising dinner for the London Consortium at Tate Modern, twisted my high heels on the sandpapery pavement and fallen hard. I cut my knee open and leaked blood and plasma for days. It didn't stop me from wearing stilettos, but ever since I have taken more care.

At the Bowery, I buy a bottle of sparkling wine and plant it on a table at the back of the room. A couple is sitting next to us. 'We met at the Breakfast Creek Hotel,' says the girl. 'This is Shane. Shane's loooovely.'

Neither of them looks comfortable. Evie starts chatting to them.

Bruce sips his bubbly. I gather he doesn't like it much. He looks wrung-out, and I know I won't last once the bottle is done. I'm a cheap drunk and a small person, and I'm already tanked. Evie will be there for as long as there's someone to talk to.

I watch Bruce, considering. *What if I take him home?* I dismiss the thought as soon as it forms. I've never asked a man home in my life. When friends have suggested it, I retort, 'What if I wake up and find out he's dumb? I won't be able to live with myself.'

'You don't have to have a conversation with them. You just show them the door.'

Bruce has stayed by my side all night. He will be lonely if I go home.

Well, why not? says that stubborn voice.

I ignore it, because the champagne has taken hold. Infected with bubbles, I want to dance again. I leap up, expecting the girl from the Breakfast Creek Hotel to come with me because she wants to get away from Shane. She remains where she is, drinking stolidly.

'I'll come.' Bruce puts down his glass.

On the dance floor beside the band, he inches close enough for me to kiss him. His hand rests in the small of my back. I take a breath and ask, 'Would you like to come home with me?'

'Do we have a choice?'

I laugh.

When I wake up the next morning, he's still asleep. My brain is jumpy with sugar from the champagne and I know I won't get back to sleep. I pick up a book from the pile beside my bed, Anita Heiss's *Tiddas*, and read until he stirs.

He doesn't leave until the afternoon. In my quiet apartment, I can hear all of his conversation. His intellect is sharp and fine. Once we start talking, we don't stop.

When I moved from London to Brisbane, I fell for the city's unabated sunshine. It dried up my depression and brought out my *joie de vivre*. I loved the winding brown river, even when it spilled its banks one summer when it wouldn't stop raining and I had English friends to stay.

'It's normally much sunnier than this!' I protested, embarrassed that it wasn't much of a change for them from England. We watched water thickening the sky, our plans for bushwalks aborted.

When I fall for Bruce, I fall harder into the city. Into the morning coffees at Café Bouquiniste in New Farm; the heat that slams into my back in summer as I run; the cycads that fan open in the City Botanic Gardens. I love anew the light slung low across Mowbray Park in late afternoons; the dark river at night as I cross it on the ferry after my French classes at Newstead; the purple thicket of jacarandas that sprawl across the sky in October; the fires of poincianas that follow. I'd forgotten what it's like to feel joy surging unexpectedly as I spoon tea leaves into a cup or collect the mail. I am a palm tree that's fruited, bursting with long, orange ropes of berries.

I Skype Oliver and tell him about Bruce. I like Skype because I can read people's lips and expressions, whereas the telephone is a constant source of anxiety.

Oliver's eyes and smile show that he's both entertained and pleased. 'There you go, Jess, it's just how it happened with Emma Woodhouse.' Oliver loves Jane Austen's *Emma* and its 1990s pop culture variant, the film *Clueless*.

'What do you mean?'

'Emma had to learn to be happy with herself before she could marry Mr Knightley.'

'You should write for the gossip pages.'

'Maybe in another life.'

We finish our conversation. I close Skype and open Facebook, another site that is a godsend. As I never phone my friends, it's easier for me to keep up with what they're doing via social media. My primary school friend Ruby, with whom I reconnected a few years ago, has posted some photos from our days at school. In one, I stand with her and my cousin Naomi, each of us wearing a Red Cross handkerchief on our heads. My grandmother, who lived down the road and who could have been a doctor had she been born half a century later, had nursed for the Red Cross during the war. She showed Naomi and me how to fold the white fabric so that the red cross rested on the centre of my forehead.

In the photo I smile frankly at the camera. My legs are locked sturdily apart, my hands clasped loosely before me. My stance and expression radiate confidence.

I'm startled by this. It makes me wonder if the anxiety of my adolescence and young adult years has coloured my recollection of my childhood.

I recall when I was eight, in Year Three. I had a crush on a boy in Year Six. On Valentine's Day at school, I made one card for my mother and another for the boy. At Friday-afternoon swimming lessons at the pool, I approached Mum, who was chatting with some other mothers, and gave her the cards.

'Thank you, darling, that's lovely. But who's this one for?'

I pointed to the boy, shading my eyes from the glare. 'Can you give it to him, please?'

The women tittered.

Even now, I remain surprised at my precociousness. Or perhaps it was simply that I was unselfconscious, like the birthmarked boy at Hanmer Springs. Or perhaps I have been that brave girl all along, and she grew into a woman who asked a man out at a bar and took him home.

Bruce lives in New Farm and I often stay at his place after I've been to French classes at Newstead. I've long wanted to learn French, largely because of a romantic notion of living in Paris to write, but also because I wasn't allowed to learn languages at school. Mum thought I would get better marks in other subjects that didn't need as much hearing. As always, I want to prove her wrong, but I find instead that she's right.

Learning French is arduous, particularly at the end of a long day. I have to strain hard to hear the liaisons, when the words run together. When I lived with Oliver in Sydney we took a term of Italian, and I can still remember more Italian words than French because the sounds are so distinct. Sometimes when I'm asked a question in French, I get flustered and reply in Italian. The class erupts with laughter, and I join in.

One evening, as I walk to Bruce's after class, passing orange bursts of trumpet creepers draped over fences, I wonder why I persist with this difficult language when I could be doing something far more natural like sign language.

I reach Bruce's gate and text him to let me in. I won't give up on French; I have promised myself that one day I'll read *Madame Bovary* in the original, but I make another mental note to look up sign language classes.

As I close my eyes that evening, exhausted after a day of work, the French class and a glass of wine, Bruce goes outside.

When he comes back in, the door creaking through my sleep, I mumble, 'Where were you?'

'Looking at the stars.'

'Why?'

'Because they're beautiful.'

I smile, pulling him to me.

I enrol in sign language classes through Deaf Services Queensland and I'm staggered, when I walk into the New Farm Neighbourhood Centre, to find nearly twenty people there. All of them have come because they're interested in learning about Deaf culture and communicating with deaf people.

An interpreter translates the teacher for our first class. My FM, after eighteen years of service, has died and I haven't yet saved enough money for a new one. I'm forced to lip-read the translator instead of watching the teacher, which is awkward, particularly after being bruised by the translator at the conference for artists with disability. We learn fingerspelling and how to have a simple conversation. It's not as difficult as French as I only have to watch, not listen.

In the second class, the translator is no longer there and I can read the teacher easily. I love the simplicity of the language and the expressiveness of her face and body. I wish that Rosa might have seen a class like this. Perhaps she might have recognised the intimacy and communion of sign language and the simple fact that, for those of us who sign, speech and writing are the same.

What would Maud have been like had she been born a century later, when the deaf community was so much stronger? Perhaps she would have grown into a winsome woman who liked collecting trinkets, who told a joke and made a person laugh, who could ride a bicycle upon the footpaths without fear. She might have learned sign language, her hands making poems in the air. She might have taught sign to her family and stayed with them, stayed 'darling Maudie', as her grandfather Thomas Murray-Prior called her. She might have sold some drawings, enough to buy a ring with a sparkling stone. She might have remained 'Birdie', her mother's pet name for her after the Bird of Paradise. She might have spread her large, lavish wings and flown.

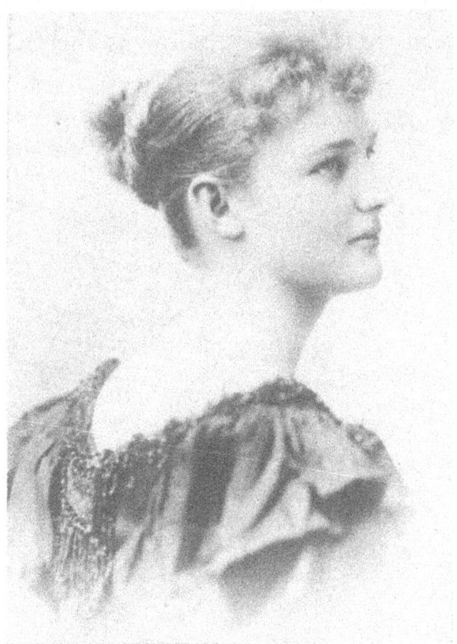

Maud in her twenties.
State Library of NSW, PXA 1403

After my class, I wave goodbye to the group who are so interested in deaf people and who are happy to learn something of us rather than make us conform. I walk back through the streets to Bruce's, listening to fruit bats screaming in the trees of New Farm Park.

Bruce opens the tall, wooden gate and kisses me, prickling my cheeks because he has forgotten to shave again. I breathe in the smell of his skin and the jasmine vine twirled around the verandah posts.

He closes the gate and leads me up the steps to the verandah, gripping my hand because of my poor balance. He leaves me on the old couch while he fetches a beer for himself and a cider for me. He sits beside me and I place a hand upon his thigh. We watch people passing on the pavement below as the Brisbane evening settles around us.

I am as close to home as I'll ever be.

Notes

1 Be/Longing

1 Frances Wilson, *Literary Seductions: Compulsive Writers and Diverted Readers*, Faber & Faber, London, 1999, p. xiv.

2 Johannes Frasnelli, Olivier Collignon, Patrice Voss and Franco Lepore, 'Crossmodal Plasticity in Sensory Loss', *Progress in Brain Research*, 2011, vol. 191, pp. 233–49.

3 Gregory D. Scott, Christina M. Karns, Mark W. Dow, Courtney Stevens and Helen J. Neville, 'Enhanced Peripheral Visual Processing in Congenitally Deaf Humans Is Supported by Multiple Brain Regions, Including Primary Auditory Cortex', *Frontiers in Human Neuroscience*, 2014, vol. 8, article no. 177.

4 Elizabeth Riddell and Yvonne Cramer, *With Fond Regards: Private Lives through Letters*, National Library of Australia, Canberra, 1995, p. 70.

5 Virginia Woolf, *A Room of One's Own and Three Guineas*, Oxford University Press, Oxford, 2015, p. 48.

6 Rosa Praed, *An Australian Heroine*, Chapman & Hall, London, 1880, p. 246.

7 ibid., p. 101.

8 Michel Foucault, 'Writing the Self', in Arnold Davidson (ed.), *Foucault and his Interlocutors*, University of Chicago Press, Chicago, 1997, p. 247.

9 ibid., p. 243.

10 Rosa Praed, *Policy and Passion: A Novel of Australian Life*, Bentley, London, 1881, p. 6

11 ibid., p. 154.

12 University of Newcastle, 'Map', *Colonial Frontier Massacres in Central and Eastern Australia 1788–1930*, c21ch.newcastle.edu.au/colonialmassacres/map.php

13 David Marr, *Patrick White: A Life*, Random House, Sydney, 2008, p. 59.

14 Rosa Praed, *An Australian Heroine*, p. 322.

15 Charlotte Brontë, *Jane Eyre*, Norton, New York, 2001, p. 93.

16 Colin Thiele, *Jodie's Journey*, Walter McVitty Books, Sydney, 1988, p. 16.

17 Rosa Praed, *Policy and Passion*, p. 91.

18 Patricia Clarke, 'Rosa Praed's Lifeline to her Australian Past', *Margin*, 2009, vol. 78, pp. 5–15, p. 6.

19 Patricia Clarke, *Rosa! Rosa! A Life of Rosa Praed, Novelist and Spiritualist*, Melbourne University Press, Melbourne, 1999, p. 23. All further citations refer to this edition.

20 ibid., p. 22.

21 ibid., pp. 42, 49.

22 ibid., p. 48.

23 ibid., p. 54.

24 ibid., pp. 10, 29, 188. Rosa is incorrectly described in many accounts as the grand-niece of Australia's first major poet, Charles Harpur. Her grandfather, Thomas Harpur, was a poet, but he was not related to Charles Harpur. See Patricia Clarke, 'The Other Harpur, or: How I Stumbled Across an Unknown Colonial Poet', *National Library of Australia News*, March 1998, pp. 18–21.

25 Rosa Praed to Nora Murray-Prior, 8 February 1878, Murray-Prior Papers, National Library of Australia (hereafter NLA), MS 7801, Box 5, Folder 33, 19/35.

26 ibid.
27 ibid.
28 ibid.
29 Case Book, Surrey History Centre, 3473/3/6, p. 437.
30 Robert J. Ruben, 'Sign Language: Its History and Contribution to the Understanding of the Biological Nature of Language', *Acta Oto-Laryngologica*, 2005, vol. 125, no. 5, pp. 464–67.
31 Brenda Jo Brueggemann, *Lend Me Your Ear: Rhetorical Constructions of Deafness*, Gallaudet University Press, Washington, DC, 1999, p. 24.
32 Harlan Lane, *When the Mind Hears: A History of the Deaf*, Random House, New York, 1984, p. 93.
33 Susan Plann, 'Pedro Ponce de Léon: Myth and Reality', in Van Clever and John Vickrey (eds), *Deaf History Unveiled: Interpretations from the New Scholarship*, Gallaudet University Press, Washington, DC, 1997, pp. 1–12.
34 Luzerne Ray, 'The Abbé de l'Épée', *American Annals of the Deaf and Dumb*, 1848, vol. 1, no. 2, pp. 69–76.
35 For more on these ideas, see Jennifer Esmail, Chapter Three, '"Human in Shape, but Only Half Human in Attributes": Sign Language, Evolutionary Theory and the Animal-Human Divide', *Reading Victorian Deafness: Signs and Sounds in Victorian Literature and Culture*, Ohio University Press, Athens, Ohio, 2013.
36 Alexander Graham Bell, *Memoir upon the Formation of a Deaf Variety of the Human Race*, National Academy of Sciences, Washington DC, 1884, p. 3.
37 ibid., p. 4.
38 H-Dirksen L. Bauman, 'Introduction: Listening to Deaf Studies', in H-Dirksen L. Bauman (ed.), *Open Your Eyes: Deaf Studies Talking*, University of Minnesota Press, Minneapolis, 2008, p. 11.
39 Donna McDonald, *The Art of Being Deaf: A Memoir*, Gallaudet University Press, Washington DC, 2014, p. 55.
40 Clarke, *Rosa! Rosa!*, p. 48.

2 Writing a Way Out

1 Patrick White, *Flaws in the Glass: A Self-Portrait*, Jonathan Cape, London, 1982, p. 15.

2 Colin Roderick, *In Mortal Bondage: The Strange Life of Rosa Praed*, Angus & Robertson, Sydney, 1948.

3 Maud Praed to Nora Murray-Prior, 24 August 1879, Murray-Prior Papers, NLA, MS 7801, Box 5, Folder 33, 19/57.

4 ibid.

5 Maud Praed to Meta and Dorothy Murray-Prior, undated (c. 1890), Murray-Prior Papers, NLA, MS 7801, Box 4, Folder 22, 16/57.

6 Maud Praed to Nora Murray-Prior, 24 August 1879, Murray-Prior Papers, NLA, MS 7801, Box 5, Folder 33, 19/57.

7 Maud Praed to Meta and Dorothy Murray-Prior, undated (c. 1890), Murray-Prior papers, NLA, MS 7801, Box 4, Folder 22, 16/57.

8 Humphrey Praed to Maud Praed, undated (c. 1898), Rosa Praed Papers, John Oxley Library, State Library of Queensland, Box 4, 4/14/27.

9 Humphrey Praed to Maud Praed, undated (c. 1898), Rosa Praed Papers, John Oxley Library, State Library of Queensland, Box 4, 4/14/25.

10 England and Wales Census, 1901.

11 D.G. Pritchard, *Education for the Handicapped: 1760–1960*, Routledge & Kegan Paul, London, 1963, p. 83.

12 H. Dominic W. Stiles, 'she had "very little ear" for speech' – ardent oralist Miss Susanna E. Hull', UCL Ear Institute & Action on Hearing Loss Libraries, 16 September 2015, blogs.ucl.ac.uk/library-rnid/2015/12/16/she-had-very-little-ear-for-speech-ardent-oralist-miss-susanna-e-hull.

13 Alexander Graham Bell, 'Prehistoric Telephone Days', *National Geographic*, 1922, vol. 61, no. 3, pp. 221–41, p. 229.

14 ibid.

15 ibid.

16 Susanna Hull, 'Do Persons Born Deaf Differ Mentally from Others who Have the Power of Hearing?', *American Annals of the Deaf and Dumb*, 1877, vol. 22, no. 4, pp. 234–40, p. 237.
17 Rosa Praed, *Fugitive Anne: A Romance of the Unexplored Bush*, John Long, London, 1902.
18 Eliza Lynn Linton to Rosa Praed, undated (c. 1897), Rosa Praed Papers, John Oxley Library, State Library of Queensland, Box 4, 4/10/22.
19 ibid.
20 Rosa Praed, *For Their Sakes*, Chapman & Hall, London, 1884, p. v.
21 Benjamin St John Ackers, 'Deaf, not Dumb' in *For Their Sakes*, Rosa Praed (ed.), Chapman & Hall, 1884, p. 44.
22 Lane, *When the Mind Hears*, p. 377.
23 Benjamin St John Ackers, 'Advantages to the Deaf of the "German" System in After Life: A Paper Written for the International Congress at Milan, September, 1880', W.H. Allen, London, 1880, p. 13.
24 Quoted in A.J. Boyce, 'Whatever Happened to Mr St. John Ackers' Deaf Daughter?' *Deaf History Journal*, 1999, vol. 3, no. 2, pp. 4–9, pp. 7–8.
25 Thomas Murray-Prior, Diary entry, Tuesday 13 June 1882, Personal diary kept on a holiday in England, 22 May – 30 August 1882, Thomas Lodge Murray-Prior papers, Mitchell Library, State Library of New South Wales, MLMSS 3117/Box 6/Item 2.
26 Lizzie Murray-Prior to Thomas Murray Prior, 7 October 1880, Murray-Prior Papers, NLA, MS 7801, Box 3, Folder 15, 12/48.
27 Lizzie Murray-Prior to Thomas Murray Prior, 27 October 1880, Murray-Prior Papers, NLA, MS 7801, Box 3, Folder 15, 12/55.
28 Elizabeth F. Boultbee, *Practical Lip-Reading for the Use of the Deaf*, L. Upcott Gill, London, 1902, p. 18.
29 Maud Praed's travel journal, Murray-Prior Papers, NLA, MS 7801, Box 6, Folder 35, 18/93.
30 Maud Praed to Thomas Murray-Prior, undated (c. 1880), Murray-Prior Papers, NLA, MS 7801, Box 3, Folder 15, 12/56.

31 Maud Praed to Dorothy Murray-Prior, Murray-Prior Papers, NLA, MS 7801, Box 5, Folder 33, 19/61.

32 For example, Maud drew an image of a punkah wallah to accompany Rosa's 'Letters from Ceylon' published on 27 April, 1895.

33 Murray-Prior Papers, NLA, MS 7801, Box 5, Folder 33, 19/63. In the State Library of New South Wales is a photograph of Rosa in this same position, and it's possible that Maud copied the image from the photograph.

34 Maud's travel journal, Murray-Prior Papers, NLA, MS 7801, Box 6, Folder 35, 18/93.

35 Maud Praed to Thomas Murray-Prior, undated (c. 1887), Murray-Prior Papers, NLA, MS 7801, Box 3, Folder 15, 12/57.

36 Clarke, *Rosa! Rosa!*, p. 136.

37 ibid.

38 Bulkley Praed to Rosa Praed, undated (c. 1893), Rosa Praed Papers, John Oxley Library, State Library of Queensland, Box 8, 8/8/11.

39 Details of this scene are taken from Bulkley Praed's letter to Rosa Praed, undated (c. 1893), Rosa-Praed Papers, John Oxley Library, State Library of Queensland, Box 8, 8/8/11.

40 Clarke, *Rosa! Rosa!*, p. 170.

41 ibid.

42 Bulkley Praed to Rosa Praed, undated (c. 1893), Rosa Praed Papers, John Oxley Library, State Library of Queensland, Box 8, 8/8/11.

43 ibid.

44 ibid.

45 Humphrey Praed to Maud Praed, undated (c. 1898), Rosa Praed Papers, John Oxley Library, State Library of Queensland, Box 4, 4/14/25.

46 Richard Noakes, 'Spiritualism, Science and the Supernatural in Mid-Victorian Britain', in Nicola Brown, Caroyln Burdett and Pamela Thurschwell (eds), *The Victorian Supernatural*, Cambridge University Press, Cambridge, 2004, p. 26.

47 Pamela Thurschwell, *Literature, Technology and Magical Thinking 1880–1920*, Cambridge University Press, Cambridge, 2001, p. 3.
48 Rosa Praed to Ruth Murray-Prior, 18 November 1929, Murray-Prior Papers, NLA, MS 7801, Box 1, Folder 10, Letter 371.
49 'Portraits of the Eighties', Rosa Praed Papers, John Oxley Library, State Library of Queensland, Box 2, 2/2/12. See also Angela Kingston's *Oscar Wilde as a Character in Victorian Fiction* (Palgrave Macmillan, Basingstoke, Hampshire, 2007) for further detail on Rosa's depictions of Wilde in her fiction.
50 'Portraits of the Eighties', Rosa Praed Papers, John Oxley Library, State Library of Queensland, Box 2, 2/2/12.
51 Maud Praed to Dorothy Murray-Prior, 7 September 1895, Murray-Prior Papers, NLA, MS 7801, Box 5, Folder 33, 19/60.
52 Bulkley Praed to Rosa Praed, 13 March 1899, Rosa Praed Papers, John Oxley Library, State Library of Queensland, Box 8, 8/8/31.
53 ibid.
54 Rosa Praed, *The Bond of Wedlock*, F.V. White and Co., London, 1887, p. 53.
55 ibid., p. 114.
56 Account of first meeting with Nancy Harward and subsequent séances, Rosa Praed Papers, John Oxley Library, State Library of Queensland, Box 1, 1/9/5.
57 Program for amateur theatricals at Kingston House, Portsmouth, 10 August 1886, Rosa Praed Papers, John Oxley Library, State Library of Queensland, Box 10, 10/10/4.
58 Andrew Lycett, *The Man Who Created Sherlock Holmes: The Life and Times of Sir Arthur Conan Doyle*, Free Press, New York, 2008, p. 34.
59 ibid.
60 ibid.
61 ibid.
62 Diary of Nancy Harward, Rosa Praed Papers, John Oxley Library, State Library of Queensland, Box 13, 13/6/1.

63 Lillian Faderman, *Surpassing the Love of Men: Romantic Friendship and Love between Women from the Renaissance to the Present*, Morrow, New York, 1981, p. 16.

64 Rosa Praed to Ruth Murray-Prior, 22 August 1928, as quoted in Clarke, *Rosa! Rosa!*, p. 168.

65 Damien Barlow, '"My Little Ghost-Slave": The Queer Lives of Rosa Praed', *Australian Literary Studies*, vol. 17, 1996, pp. 344–52.

66 Rosa Praed, *Nyria*, T. Fisher Unwin, London, 1904, p. 3.

67 ibid.

68 ibid., p. 4.

69 Account of first meeting with Nancy Harward and subsequent séances, Rosa Praed Papers, John Oxley Library, State Library of Queensland, Box 1, 1/9/5.

70 Terry Castle, *The Apparitional Lesbian: Female Homosexuality and Modern Culture*, Columbia University Press, New York, 1993, p. 30. Castle's italics.

71 Maud Praed to Thomas Murray-Prior, undated (c. 1890), Murray-Prior Papers, NLA, MS 7801, Box 3, Folder 17, 15/55.

72 Maud Praed to Thomas Murray-Prior, undated (c. 1887), Murray-Prior Papers, NLA, MS 7801, Box 3, Folder 15, 12/57.

73 Bulkley Praed to Rosa Praed, 13 March 1899, Rosa Praed Papers, John Oxley Library, State Library of Queensland, Box 8, 8/8/31.

74 Maud Praed to Nora Murray-Prior, undated (c. 1888), Murray-Prior Papers, NLA, MS 7801, Box 5, Folder 33, 19/59.

75 Maud Praed to Nora Murray-Prior, 24 August 1877, Murray-Prior Papers, NLA, MS 7801, Box 5, Folder 33, 19/57.

76 Maud Praed to Meta and Dorothy Murray-Prior, undated (c. 1890), Murray Prior Papers, NLA, MS 7801, Box 4, Folder 22, 16/57.

77 Bulkley Praed to Rosa Praed, 13 March 1899, Rosa Praed Papers, John Oxley Library, State Library of Queensland, Box 8, 8/8/31.

78 Maud Praed to Thomas Murray-Prior, undated (c. 1887), Murray-Prior Papers, NLA, MS 7801, Box 3, Folder 15, 12/57.

79 Humphrey Praed to Maud Praed, 7 November 1904, Rosa Praed Papers, John Oxley Library, State Library of Queensland, Box 4, 4/15/35.

80 Humphrey Praed to Maud Praed, 7 November 1904, Rosa Praed Papers, John Oxley Library, State Library of Queensland, Box 4, 4/15/35.

81 Humphrey Praed to Rosa Praed, 24 November 1901, Rosa Praed Papers, John Oxley Library, State Library of Queensland, Box 4, 4/15/18.

82 'Death of Mr Campbell Praed', *Northampton Mercury*, no. 9437, 8 November 1901, p 7.

83 Humphrey Praed to Rosa Praed, 24 November 1901, Rosa Praed Papers, John Oxley Library, State Library of Queensland, Box 4, 4/15/18.

84 'Funeral of Mr Campbell Praed', *Northampton Mercury*, no. 9437, 8 November 1901, p. 5.

85 Case Book, Surrey History Centre, 3473/3/6, p. 437.

86 Susan Sidlauskas, 'Inventing the Medical Portrait: Photography at the "Benevolent Asylum" of Holloway, c. 1885–1889', *Medical Humanities*, 2013, vol. 39, no. 1, pp. 29–37, p. 32.

87 *The Builder*, 7 January 1882.

88 Julia Nurse, 'Holloway Sanatorium for the Insane', Wellcome Library Blog, 8 July 2016, blog.wellcomelibrary.org/2016/07/holloway-sanatorium-for-the-insane.

89 Sidlauskas, 'Inventing the Medical Portrait', p. 32.

90 Rosa Praed to Louise Chandler Moulton, 1 March [1904] Louise Chandler Moulton Papers, National Library of Congress, MSS33787, Box 34, Microfilm Reel 10.

91 Case Book, Surrey History Centre, 3473/3/6, p. 437.

92 Details taken from Humphrey Praed's letter to Rosa Praed, 18 December 1902, Rosa Praed Papers, John Oxley Library, State Library of Queensland, Box 8, 8/8/44.

93 Humphrey Praed to Rosa Praed, Rosa Praed Papers, 18 December 1902, John Oxley Library, State Library of Queensland, Box 8, 8/8/44.
94 Case Book, Surrey History Centre, 3473/3/6, p. 437.
95 Bulkley Praed to Rosa Praed, 15 December 1902, Rosa Praed Papers, John Oxley Library, State Library of Queensland, Box 8, 8/8/45.
96 Case Book, Surrey History Centre, 3473/3/6, p. 437.
97 ibid.
98 Bulkley Praed to Rosa Praed, 13 April 1905, Rosa Praed Papers, John Oxley Library, State Library of Queensland, Box 8, 8/8/65.
99 Bulkley Praed to Rosa Praed, 25 July 1904, Rosa Praed Papers, John Oxley Library, State Library of Queensland, Box 8, 8/8/58.
100 Bulkley Praed to Rosa Praed, 13 April 1905, Rosa Praed Papers, John Oxley Library, State Library of Queensland, Box 8, 8/8/65.
101 Humphrey Praed to Rosa Praed, 10 January 1903, Rosa Praed Papers, John Oxley Library, State Library of Queensland, Box 4, 4/15/24.
102 Humphrey Praed to Rosa Praed, 11 July 1903, Rosa Praed Papers, John Oxley Library, State Library of Queensland, Box 4, 4/15/26.
103 Case Book, Surrey History Centre, 3473/3/6, p. 437.
104 See Anna Shepherd, *Institutionalizing the Insane in Nineteenth-Century England*, Pickering and Chatto, London, 2014.
105 Brenda Jo Brueggemann, *Deaf Subjects: Between*, New York University Press, New York, 2009, pp. 117–40.
106 Graeme Gooday and Karen Sayer, *Managing the Experience of Hearing Loss in Britain, 1830–1930*, Palgrave Macmillan, Basingstoke, Hampshire, 2017, pp. 55–59.
107 Typescript headed 'Account of Luncheon Party Where I Met the Prince of Wales in Cannes – a Few Months After the Publication of "Nadine"', Rosa Praed Papers, John Oxley Library, State Library of Queensland, Box 2, 2/2/18.
108 Andrew Solomon, *Far From the Tree: Parents, Children and the Search for Identity*, Random House, London, 2012.
109 Rosa Praed to Dorothy Murray-Prior, 13 July 1924, Murray-Prior Papers, NLA, MS 7801, Box 1, Folder 5, Letter 172.

110 Rosa Praed to Nora Murray-Prior, 29 April 1917, Murray-Prior Papers, NLA, MS 7801, Box 1, Folder 2, Letter 42.
111 Rosa Praed to Dorothy Murray-Prior, 13 July 1924, Murray-Prior Papers, NLA, MS 7801, Box 1, Folder 5, Letter 172.
112 Rosa Praed, *An Australian Heroine*, p. 342.
113 Rosa Praed, *Zéro: A Story of Monte Carlo*, Chapman & Hall, London, 1884. p. 131.
114 Rosa Praed, *Madame Izàn: A Tourist Story*, Chatto & Windus, London, 1899, p. 264.
115 Jacques Rancière, *Mute Speech: Literature, Critical Theory, and Politics*, trans. James Swenson, Columbia University Press, New York, 2011.
116 Rosa Praed to Dorothy Murray-Prior, 13 July 1924, Murray-Prior Papers, NLA, MS 7801, Box 1, Folder 5, Letter 172.
117 McDonald, *The Art of Being Deaf*, pp. 13–14.
118 Rosa Praed, *The Romance of a Station*, Trischler, London, 1889, p. 3.
119 ibid., p. 10.
120 ibid., p. 10.
121 Clarke, *Rosa! Rosa!*, p. 35.
122 Rosa Praed Papers, John Oxley Library, State Library of Queensland, Box 3, 3/7/3.
123 Clarke, *Rosa! Rosa!*, p. 36.
124 Pamela Thurschwell, *Literature, Technology and Magical Thinking, 1880–1920*, p. 106.
125 Rosa Praed, *The Romance of a Station*, p. 74.
126 ibid., p. 75.
127 Tom Standage, *The Victorian Internet: The Remarkable Story of the Telegraph and the Nineteenth Century's On-line Pioneers*, Berkley Books, 1999.
128 Cited in Douglas C. Baynton, '"A Silent Exile on this Earth": The Metaphorical Construction of Deafness in the Nineteenth Century', *American Quarterly*, vol. 44, no. 2, 1992, pp. 216–43, pp. 221–22.
129 Clarke, *Rosa! Rosa!*, p. 243.
130 Oliver Sacks, *Seeing Voices: A Journey into the World of the Deaf*, Pan Books, London, 1991, p. 126. See also 'History Behind DPN:

What Happened…', Gallaudet University, www.gallaudet.edu/about/history-and-traditions/deaf-president-now/the-issues/history-behind-dpn.

131 Donald Moores, 'Partners in Progress: The 21st International Congress on Education of the Deaf and the Repudiation of the 1880 Congress of Milan', *American Annals of the Deaf*, 2010, vol. 155, no. 3, pp. 309–10.

132 Murray-Prior Papers, MS 7801, detailed inventory, Appendix 2.

3 Reading Hearts

1 Brueggemann, *Lend Me Your Ear*, p. 8.

2 Rosa Praed, *My Australian Girlhood: Sketches and Impressions of Bush Life*, T. Fisher Unwin, London, 1902, p. 4.

3 Rosa Praed, *Fugitive Anne*, p. 46.

4 Andrew McCann, 'Unknown Australia: Rosa Praed's Vanished Race', *Australian Literary Studies*, vol. 22, 2005, pp. 37–50, p. 49.

5 Jennifer Esmail, *Reading Victorian Deafness*, p. 193.

6 ibid., p. 201.

7 Brueggemann, *Lend Me Your Ear*, pp. 50–51.

8 Lennard J. Davis, *Enforcing Normalcy Disability, Deafness, and the Body*, Verso, London, 1995, p. 24.

9 ibid., p. 26.

10 ibid., pp. 29–30.

11 ibid., p. 10.

12 James Woodward and Thomas P. Horejes, 'deaf/Deaf: Origins and Usage', *The SAGE Deaf Studies Encyclopedia*, SAGE Publications, Thousand Oaks, California, 2016, pp. 285–87.

13 Brueggemann, *Lend Me Your Ear*, p. 152.

14 Ellen Samuels, 'My Body, My Closet: Invisible Disability and the Limits of Coming-Out Discourse', *GLQ: A Journal of Lesbian and Gay Studies*, 2003, vol. 9, pp. 233–55, p. 247.

15 ibid., pp. 241, 242.

16 Clarke, *Rosa! Rosa!*, p. 198.

17 Helen Sword, *Ghostwriting Modernism*, Cornell University Press, Ithaca, New York, 2002, pp. 13–14.
18 Peter Fripp, *The Book of Johannes*, Rider & Co., London, 1945, p. 12.
19 Details are taken from Rosa Praed Papers, John Oxley Library, State Library of Queensland, Box 7, 7/11/1.
20 ibid., Box 12, 12/6/1.
21 ibid.
22 ibid.
23 Rosa Praed, Typescript on different incarnations of Praed and Harward, Rosa Praed Papers, John Oxley Library, State Library of Queensland, Box 1A, 1A/5/1.
24 Clarke, *Rosa! Rosa!*, p. 203.
25 Rosa Praed to Dorothy and Ruth Murray-Prior, 3 February 1931, Letter 407, Murray-Prior Papers, NLA, MS 7801, Box 1, Folder 11.
26 Diary, 1930–1931, with records of mediumistic conversations with Nancy Harward and others, Rosa Praed Papers, John Oxley Library, State Library of Queensland, Box 7, 7/7/1.
27 Frederic W.H. Myers to Rosa Praed, 27 June 1884, Rosa Praed Papers, John Oxley Library, State Library of Queensland, Box 8, 8/1/9.
28 William Crookes to Rosa Praed 21 May 1904, Rosa Praed Papers, John Oxley Library, State Library of Queensland, Box 8, 8/4/4.
29 Rosa Praed to Ruth and Dorothy Murray-Prior, 9 June 1932, Murray-Prior Papers, NLA, MS 7801, Box 5, Folder 33, 19/49.
30 Rosa Praed, *Lady Bridget in the Never-Never Land: A Story of Australian Life*, Hutchinson, London, 1915, p. 481.
31 Maud Praed to Dorothy Murray-Prior, undated (c. 1896), Murray-Prior Papers, NLA, MS 7801, Box 5, Folder 33, 19/61.
32 Maud Praed's travel journal, Murray-Prior Papers, NLA, MS 7801, Box 6, Folder 35, 18/93.
33 Humphrey Praed to Rosa Praed, 18 December 1902, Rosa Praed Papers, John Oxley Library, State Library of Queensland, Box 8, 8/8/44.

34 Edmund Gurney, Frederic Myers and Frank Podmore, *Phantasms of the Living*, vol. I, Trübner and Co., London, 1886, p. xxxv.

35 Donna McDonald, *The Art of Being Deaf*, p. 19.

36 ibid., p. 11.

37 Michael Davidson, *Concerto for the Left Hand: Disability and the Defamiliar Body*, University of Michigan Press, Ann Arbor, 2008, p. 4.

38 Margaret Atwood, *Negotiating with the Dead: A Writer on Writing*, Cambridge University Press, Cambridge, 2002, p. 34.

39 ibid., pp. 178–79.

Acknowledgements

I left for London to research this book nearly fifteen years ago, and along the way I collected numerous people to help with its creation. Thank you to:

The University of Melbourne for its provision of the Sir Arthur Sims Travelling Scholarship, which made it possible for me to undertake my PhD in London and start my research. I am also grateful to Arts Queensland for an Individuals Grant, which enabled me to continue my research in Australia.

Dr Louise D'Arcens, for introducing me to the *pharmakon*. Dr Ian Henderson, for his kindness and support during my time in London and for his comments, together with those of Professor Steven Connor and Professor Gail Jones, on the earliest iterations of this work.

Catherine Sharp, for her friendship in London and the years after, and for helping with my research on return visits.

My second family in England, Pia and Jamie, for taking a homesick Australian under their wing while I lived in London, and for hosting me on return trips. Lou and Matt, for providing warmth and nourishment on my stints in Canberra.

Dr Jill Ashburner, for her generosity and flexibility while I worked on this book and other writing projects, and for introducing me to Dr Donna McDonald.

Donna, for being my touchstone. Her understanding and friendship guided me towards my deaf self, and this book would never have evolved without her prompting.

Scholars who paved the way for this work, particularly Dr Chris Tiffin and Dr Patricia Clarke. Rosa Praed's archives are vast, and without their research I would have had a much harder time of carrying out mine.

Staff at the many wonderful libraries and archives I consulted for my work, including the National Library of Australia, the John Oxley Library, Woking Library and the British Library. In particular, Dominic Stiles of the UCL Ear Institute and Action on Hearing Loss Library, London.

My publisher Terri-ann White for having faith in this book; Nicola Young for her careful, considerate editing; and the wonderful team at UWAP for turning my words into a beautiful object. My agent Pippa Masson for her ongoing dedication to bringing my work into the world.

My fellow writers for aiding my apprenticeship in non-fiction and for providing critical feedback: Inga Simpson, Michelle Dicinoski, Melissa Fagan, Kris Olsson and the Bright Boats group. I also appreciate the insights and knowledge of Amanda Tink.

My teachers, Tony Muller and Jennifer Woolcott. My audiologist, Dr John Pearcy, for helping me to hear in my life and at work. Dr John Rooney, who saved my life at Tamworth Hospital (and who later opened a bookstore).

Bella, for always making sure I was heard and, together with her husband, for putting a roof over my head when I moved to Brisbane. Mum and Dad, for the other roof, and for their tireless encouragement of my writing. Oliver, as always, for being my other ear, my best friend and an amazing and generous brother, and for rescuing me from the cassowary in Far North Queensland. And Bruce, for the love and jokes, and for opening up my life in unexpected ways.

Parts of this work were recognised by a shortlisting in the *Australian Book Review* Calibre Prize and have been published in *Meanjin*, *Southerly*, *Cordite*, *Sydney Review of Books*, *Journal of the Association for the Study of Australian Literature*, *New Scholar* and *Hecate*. Litmags and scholarly journals are the lifeblood of Australian literature, and I am grateful to these literary outlets for publishing our writing.

I acknowledge the Jagera and Turrbal people on whose country this book was written, and the Kamilaroi people on whose country I grew up, and I recognise their ongoing connection to their lands.